Anatomy, Stretching
& Training for Cyclists

Anatomy, Stretching & Training for Cyclists

A Step-by-Step Guide to Getting the Most from Your Bicycle Workouts

Lisa Purcell

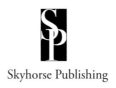

Skyhorse Publishing

CONTENTS

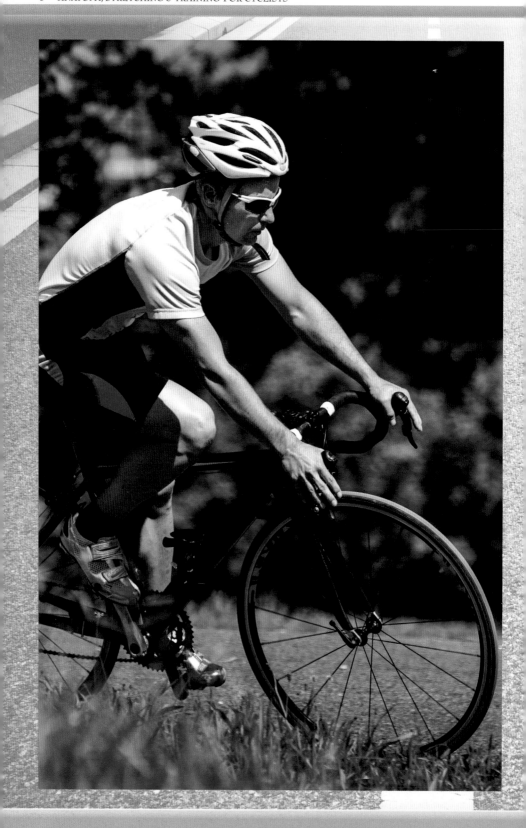

INTRODUCTION: FIT FOR CYCLING

As a cyclist, you already know how wonderful a bike ride can make your body feel. During a good ride, your legs are pumping, your abdominal muscles are engaged, and a wide spectrum of different muscle groups are working hard as you power forward.

But you can feel even better. When it comes to optimizing performance, avoiding aches and pains, and generally enhancing how you feel while cycling, there is always room for improvement. This book will give you all the tools you need to condition your body to make every ride your best one.

Whether you are a beginner or a seasoned athlete, you can benefit from stretches that limber up tight muscles, strengthening moves that target your core and lower body, and exercises that improve your posture and hone the sense of balance that is so vital to cycling effectively. The exercises in these pages are designed to work a wide range of muscles that come into play when cycling. They can be performed in your living room, so that in between forays into the streets or along the mountain trails, you will be working your entire body to meet the unique demands of your sport.

CYCLING BASICS

CYCLING IS AN INCREDIBLY REWARDING activity. With its low impact on the joints and high rate of calorie burn, it is a great choice for anyone wanting to get (and stay) in shape. It is also accessible to enthusiasts of all fitness levels: no matter what your capability when beginning or returning to the sport, cycling allows for all forms of progression, from riding a flat mile in the local park loop to completing your first hilly 100-mile endurance ride.

One sport, many benefits

The sport of cycling carries fantastic health benefits. It has been known to boost mental health, decrease the risk of coronary heart disease, and improve coordination skills. Studies have connected cycling to not only the physical effects of decreased waistlines and prolonged caloric burn, but also to heightened emotional health, mental capacity, and even earning potential and productivity at work.

Getting back on your bike

If you're reading this book, you likely already have some level of interest in cycling. Perhaps you've seen the enviable chiseled quadriceps and calves of professional cyclists riding the Tour de France or maybe you're looking for a low-impact transition from running. Maybe you want to try racing and are looking to increase speed and power output. If you're a triathlete, you may be seeking to transfer your current skills and capabilities to the cycling portion

of your racing. Some of you may want to embark on a fitness regimen that also benefits the environment, choosing to bike to work rather than drive a car. Or, you may simply love riding a bike and want to get better at it.

Whatever the nature of your interest in cycling, this book will help you to get fit and stay fit for the physical demands of the sport. This is accomplished through targeting the muscles predominantly used to bring about forward motion of the bike, as well as through building the powerhouse muscles that will ultimately lead to a toned and balanced cycling body. After all, cycling is not all about the legs, but about core strength, balance, posture, and flexibility too.

Cyclists should be well-rounded athletes, recognizing that strength on the bike draws from all the body's major and minor muscle groups. In the following pages, illustrations accompanying the step-by-step instructions will show you exactly which muscles you are working.

Retool your equipment

As you start out on a cycling program, it's likely you'll experience some muscle soreness, especially in the back, knees, and neck, or even wrists and hands if the bike you're using was never properly fitted to your body. The good news is that as long as your bike's frame is the right size (a reputable bike shop can help you determine this), it is possible to adjust your body position so you do

Choose your terrain

Starting out cycling or returning to the sport you loved as a child can be as simple as getting the bike in your garage tuned up and then heading out for a spin. Nonetheless, we all have different tolerances and capabilities when it comes to riding in vehicular traffic, and if you are not used to cycling, go first to a bike path or some other safe location before riding in the street. It is important to get comfortable with starting and stopping, scanning and signaling, and feeling the leaning and turning effects that come about when you cycle. Initially, if you stay at a reasonably low speed on flat terrain, you are unlikely to experience muscle fatigue; after all, the bike is an incredibly efficient machine.

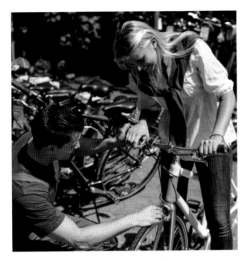

not feel aches and pains. Always give as much specific information as you can on what is hurting your body and where; front-of-the-knee pain determines a different adjustment than back-of-the-knee pain, for example.

GETTING YOUR BIKE IN SHAPE

If you haven't ridden your bike in a year or more, before going out for that first ride, put your bike in the car and head first to your local bike shop and have a qualified mechanic give it a tune-up.

Because the bike is a complex machine with many moving and integrated parts, there is an increased risk of injury when using a bicycle that is not in proper working order. Even if you're mechanically inclined, there are many subtle and not so subtle adjustments an experienced mechanic will make that will not only improve your overall experience on the bike, but will also increase your speed and efficiency. It's relatively easy to recognize a flat tire, but far less easy to determine a loose and dangerous bottom bracket or head tube. And many components on new bikes have very specific tensions or torques where

overtightening could lead to dangerous failure or cause stress cracks and fractures.

Depending on the condition and age of your bike, expect to pay approximately $50 to $125 for a professional tune-up, which can include an overall inspection, as well as adjusting or replacing cables and housing; cleaning of the frame, cassette, chain, and cogs; lubricating the chain; adjusting the shifting and braking abilities; and replacing brake pads, handlebar tape, and cracked and worn tires.

A tune-up typically takes a few days, and it should never be overlooked. Care will also be given to the use of lubricants specifically designed for bike parts; a common household lubricant like WD-40 is neither intended for nor useful in cycling applications.

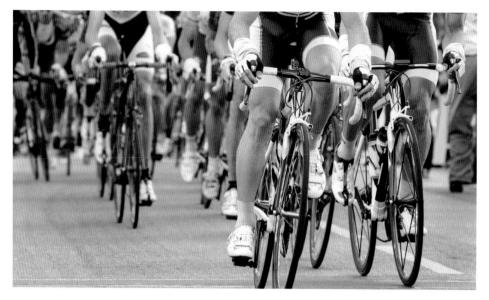

Improving cycling performance

Cycling fitness is determined largely by strength, cardiovascular endurance, muscle endurance, and power. Natural ability plays a role, but a well-trained, well-developed body can achieve even the most ambitious of goals. Whether you're a beginning cyclist or a Cat 1 racer, starting with a deep understanding of the body's interconnectedness is the first step in achieving objectives. Simply riding more miles, or faster miles, will not necessarily lead to a continuous improvement in fitness. It's more important to take a well-reasoned approach to your body's strengths and weaknesses, which in turn will allow you to craft a fitness plan that works for you.

Many areas of fitness can play a role in a cyclist's performance. Perhaps a beginner's goal is simply to complete a long ride, whatever that total mileage may be. Perhaps a competitive racer's goal is to have greater power output. A super-busy mother may want to pack as much intensity as possible into her short exercise sessions. With their targeted approach, the exercises in this book will prove effective for any cyclist of any level who wants to develop endurance (whether cardiovascular or muscular), speed, and power.

It is a common misconception that cycling fitness is centered on the lower body: the quadriceps, hamstrings, and calves. Naturally, the muscles in these groups produce a bike's forward motion, but development of the body as a whole will lead to balance, injury avoidance, and sustainability. After all, few people enter the sport of cycling thinking it's for a short time. With proper muscle development and care, cycling is a sport that can and should be enjoyed well into your golden years. In fact, French cyclist Robert Marchand just set a record time for a 100-year-old when he rode 62 miles at a velodrome in Lyon.

A well-balanced approach

Whether you're a beginner cyclist or have been riding for years, you already know that in order to ride a bike, you need to balance. Lean the bike too far one way or the other and you'll likely find yourself falling. Failing to balance your body can lead to the same effect— an inability to keep cycling in the way you wish to cycle.

Be careful not to let your training become too one-sided. The repetitive position and mechanics of cycling can lead to imbalance in the body's development, and just like you will at some point consider upgrading your gear, it's important to consider upgrading your body's focus to include exercises that develop your body as a whole.

The proper development of your musculature and sene of balance will ensure that your new or long-

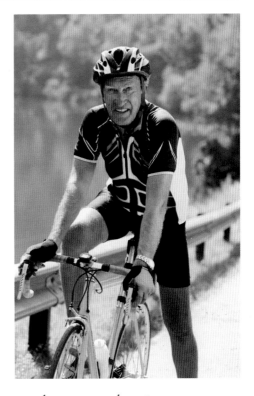

standing interest doesn't give way to abandonment of the sport because you've developed chronic-use injuries or unmitigated aches and pains.

Avoiding chronic-use injuries

Have you ever sat hunched over your computer for an entire day? When you finally rise, the stretch that makes you feel better counteracts the forward hunch. Maybe you lean, arms open, stretching back over your chair with your neck extended. Even if you are not feeling pronounced discomfort, it often feels natural to counteract a prolonged body position by moving in the other direction. Too much of anything can lead to stress and strain.

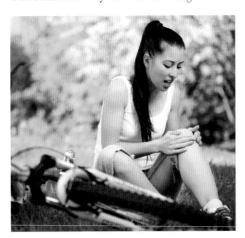

Cycling is not unique in this respect. In other sports, where running, jumping, catching, or stretching are carried out over and over, different chronic-use injuries are common. For instance, a tennis player may experience tendonitis in the elbow, while a basketball player may feel knee pain from running and jumping. In sports, the most common forms of injury involve the knees, neck, and back.

In cycling, discomfort can happen for many reasons. When you first start cycling, or begin again after a long break, some initial muscle soreness is normal, and often goes away with time. An improperly fitting bike can also cause discomfort, as can sitting in an uncomfortable position on the bike. But beyond these factors, repetitive motion is a major cause of imbalance and injury for cyclists.

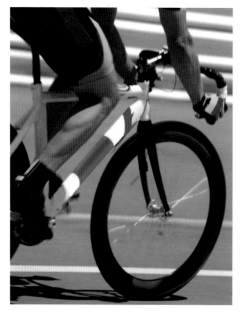

Pedaling calls for repeated flexion, a bending movement that decreases the angle between two parts, and extension, a straightening that increases the angle. When pedaling a bike, for example, the leg moving downward is flexing at the knee and hip while the leg moving upward is extending at the knee and hip. Both the knee and hip areas are therefore common sites of chronic-use injuries, such as patellar tendonitis, bursitis, iliotibial band syndrome, hip bursitis, hip flexor strains, and snapping hip syndrome.

Adduction versus abduction

Based on their characteristics of adduction versus abduction, the exercises in this book specifically address how to counteract the negative effects of the repetitive flexion and extension motions associated with riding a bike. Simply put, abduction is a motion that pulls a limb or other bodily structure away from the body—using your deltoids to raise your arm away from the side of your body, for example. Adduction pulls a structure toward the body, as in squeezing your inner thighs together using your adductor longus muscles.

Utilizing a careful balance of strength and flexibility, abduction and adduction will lead to optimal cycling performance. Also, specifically choosing exercises such as the Spinal Twist (page 36) and the Bilateral Seated Forward Bend (page 38) will target opposite motions as experienced on a bike.

Gearing up

Other than the bike itself, cycling requires no special equipment or clothing. Although in many areas, helmets are law, in many places you can literally just get on your bike and go. Still, to add comfort and injury protection, think about gearing up with some cycling-specific extras.

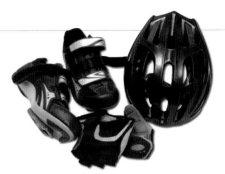

Helmet: Protecting your head is essential, which is why helmets are mandated by law in many places. If you fall, the right helmet can spare you from brain injury—and even save your life. Look for a sleek lightweight design of high-impact-withstanding material that is ventilated to keep your head cool. Moisture-wicking pads can help control sweat, too. Your helmet should fit your head easily with no pinching.

Shorts and pants: Long hours in the saddle can be hard on your nether regions, so think about getting yourself some padded biking shorts or pants. Most are made of lycra with moisture-wicking chamois padding, which makes for a far more comfortable ride.

Jerseys and windbreakers: Again made of moisture-wicking fabric, a cycling jersey makes riding more comfortable. Look for designs with back pockets for easy storage that won't impede your movements and drop-tail hems that are longer in the back so that they don't ride up. When you cycle in changeable weather, tuck a foldable windbreaker into your jersey pocket. Try a drop-tail design made from water-resistant and windproof fabric. For both jerseys and windbreakers, go for bright colors, which makes it easy for motorists to see you on the road.

Gloves: Adding a layer of padding under your palms and thumb beds can protect your hands. To avoid hand discomfort, numbness, and fatigue, look for padded fingerless sport gloves.

Sunglasses: Photochromatic sunglasses that adapt to changing light conditions are a cycling essentials, protecting your eyes from sun and wind. Sunglasses should fit snugly but comfortably—you don't want them flying off mid-ride. Look for shatterproof plastic with cutouts for ventilation.

CYCLING SHOES

If you ride regularly, a good pair of cycling shoes is a worthy investment. You can ride a bike in just about any shoes, but anyone who rides regularly can benefit from shoes designed specifically for bicycling. Many designs are available, depending on purpose—whether road, mountain, touring, competition, or casual riding. Cycling shoes should be rigid, which transfers power from cyclist to pedal more efficiently than a soft shoe. Some models are equipped with an attachment system that grips the shoe firmly to the pedal.

Cycling and nutrition

It's a common cycling adage to eat before you're hungry and drink before you're thirsty, and as a general rule this serves a valuable purpose. Because cycling is an endurance sport, it is critical to keep your body fueled. It is crucial to begin your workout hydrated and to stay that way throughout. Though experts disagree on the amount of fluids to be consumed during a workout, there is no disagreement that lack of proper hydration will lead to a dramatic decrease in ability and performance.

Nutrition is a science and a subject worthy of an entire book. People will choose foods for a variety of reasons while they cycle. Some choices are made based on sound scientific principles of glycogen stores and uptake rates, while others will be made based on the

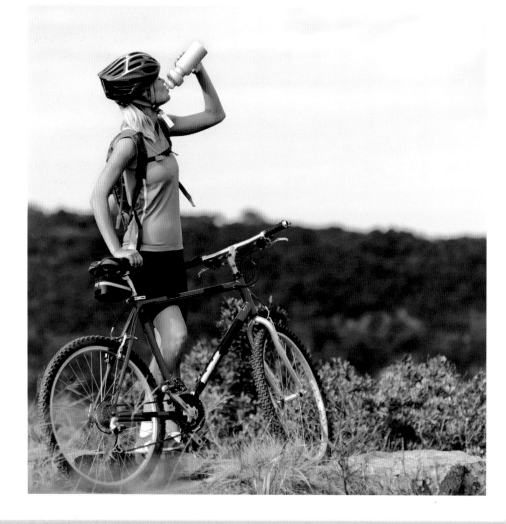

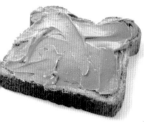

body's tolerance for certain ingredients when under stress. There are supplements and easily convertible carbohydrate sports gels, or there are simple peanut butter sandwiches. The choice is personal and is best found through trial and error for your own goals.

Beginners often hold a common misconception concerning how much to eat during a ride, assuming they must fuel up for every outing. Generally, if you're going out for only an hour, don't stop for a calorie-rich peanut butter sandwich along the way. The body can store about 90 minutes worth of fuel to use. If your ride will be shorter than that, it's not necessary to be overly concerned with consuming calories or downing endurance drinks.

It can be easily said, though, that while riding distances, you should be consuming carbohydrates. The body will extract glucose from carbohydrates much more easily than from protein or fat, so a pre-ride choice of high-fat cream cheese on your bagel will only serve to make you feel sluggish. The body will be working hard to get the glucose out of the fat while it works easily getting it from dried fruit or just a plain bagel.

A good rule of thumb is to consume carbohydrates every 30 minutes while on a prolonged ride, even if you're not feeling hungry. If you choose to use a sports gel, remember to drink plenty of water when you consume it. Cheaper than sports gels is the simple jelly bean. It's easy to digest, high in carbohydrates, and simple to eat while riding.

Eating before you're hungry and drinking before you're thirsty are good rules to follow while riding, but what about after your ride? The first 30 minutes after your ride are absolutely critical to replenishing glycogen stores. Some experts recommend taking your weight and dividing that figure in half to determine the number of carbohydrate grams you should consume in this narrow post-ride window. The window for replenishing these stores is literally only 30 to 60 minutes, so make sure to have recovery foods readily available. An excellent and scientifically sound choice for post-ride consumption is low-fat chocolate milk. It's rich in carbohydrates and protein, which are needed to help refuel and repair muscles. Again, it should be consumed ideally within the first 30 minutes after finishing your cycling workout.

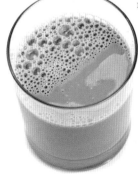

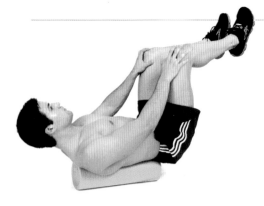

Your home gym

All of the exercises in this book balance the body and optimize performance, but also facilitate working out at home with minimal specialty equipment. Equipment used throughout the book consists of the following:

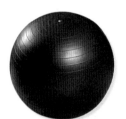

- a mat
- a chair
- a small medicine ball
- a large Swiss ball
- a small roller
- a large roller

You may find that it helps to designate an area of your home as a workout space. As much as possible, try to keep the space free of clutter and other distractions. It is all too easy to get caught up in thinking about phone calls you need to make, e-mails you need to return, and so on. But if you devote time to getting stronger and more flexible, you'll come to understand that the benefits merit the time spent away from your cell phone. Exercising on a regular schedule helps to turn your home workout into a habit; even 15 minutes three times per week will go a long way toward improving your overall fitness—and, in turn, your experience and performance on the bike.

How to use this book

In the following pages, you will find a wide variety of exercises, all selected to benefit you as a cyclist. Flexibility is vital, and the first section describes how to stretch your neck, your feet, and pretty much everything in between. You'll then move on to exercises that strengthen your legs and arms in preparation for the demands of cycling; many exercises in this section work other parts of the body as well.

Next, you'll find an array of exercises to strengthen your core. This is that powerhouse of muscles, including the abdominals, hip adductors, spinal extensors, and more, from which all bodily movement originates. And finally, you'll find moves that hone your posture, sense of balance, and coordination.

Follow the step-by-step photos and instructions to ensure correct form. To get a sense of which muscles you are targeting, review the anatomical illustrations that highlight the visible working muscles. Lists of target muscles, benefits, and conditions that preclude certain exercises will enable you to choose a set of exercises that works best for your own needs. Tips on performing the exercises correctly and advice on what to avoid will help you get the most from your workout.

SPINNING VERSUS CYCLING

Spin, or spinning, is a form of indoor exercise offered in many gyms. It is generally a group class with participants on exercise or stationary bikes. The kind of bikes can vary greatly, but usually are adjustable in many capacities and can include special pedals to accommodate clip-in cycling shoes.

Spinning's intense, sweat-producing workout and weather-benign indoor atmosphere has led to its surge of popularity among cyclists and fitness enthusiasts. Many cyclists struggle to maintain their fitness through the winter when poor road conditions or lack of cold-weather gear keeps them off the bike for months at a time. Though cycling outdoors in winter can be enjoyable and safe, many people are not willing to manage the potentially (but not necessarily) substantial cost of special gear or the possibility of ice.

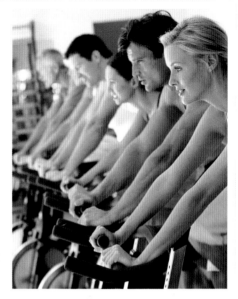

A typical spin class includes a pack of bikes facing one instructor's bike, often with high-decibel motivating music, and frequently occurs with the lights dimmed or at times turned off altogether. Because the bikes are not actually moving anywhere, the instructor will often use a microphone to describe the "ride" for participants: imagery of flats, mountains, coasts, or especially beautiful scenery is invoked as bike tension is repeatedly self-altered to simulate hills, sprints, easy spinning, and recovery. Often the instructor, specifically trained in this kind of workout, will have participants sit and spin at a given pace (usually to the beat of the music), or will call for standing and pedaling or any given combination thereof.

When given an authentic effort, this workout can be intensely sweat-producing and exhausting, often a welcome effect in the cold of winter. The benefits naturally include development of cardiac capability and quadriceps strength. Care should be taken, however, to recognize that spinning is not necessarily a good mimic of actual cycling. There is no balance employed, no true navigation of terrain, and at times the muscle-fatigue techniques of hovering over the seat by just a few inches is not comparable to the action that takes place on an actual bike. Additionally, the classes are often taught by trainers who are not cyclists, and while seeking to provide a good workout, they do not always provide a workout that benefits cycling goals.

If you're considering taking a spin class, also consider wearing actual cycling gear; padded shorts can contribute a good deal towards comfort on the often-hard saddles of stationary bikes.

For people who are interested in increasing their performance specifically in spin class, the exercises dedicated to strength and leg training will help develop optimal performance. Wall Sit (page 86), Thigh Rock-Back (page 100), and Power Squat (page 144), for example, are excellent choices for building strong legs. As with cycling outdoors, however, great care should be placed on developing balance in the body. Spin is a repetitive motion and it's possible to develop over-use injuries. Hip Flexor Stretch (page 48), Hip/Iliotibial Band Stretch (page 50), and Hand-to-Toe Lift (page 64) and will be especially helpful in counteracting the motion of spin.

CYCLING EQUIPMENT

THERE ARE AS MANY DIFFERENT kinds of bicycles as there are reasons for riding them. Bike types can be divided by function or sport. Though it's certainly possible to achieve health benefits from riding any kind of bike, most riders choose a mountain or road bike for fitness. Advanced riders, who like to compete, go for the specialty designs, such as cyclocross bikes and track bikes.

The differences between the many kinds of bikes on the market are primarily in the geometry of the frame design, materials used, and the kinds of tires that suit different terrains.

Beginners may feel more stable if they choose a bicycle with a more upright geometry, or one that allows them to put a foot flat on the ground without having to come off the saddle.

If you opt for your first mountain bike after riding a road bike for years, as you increase the number of miles you're riding on pavement you will notice the thicker, knobbier tires of a mountain bike create a lot of rolling resistance. Road bikes, with their thin tires, roll faster than the thicker mountain bike tires, but are more delicate.

Know your needs

To determine which kind of bike is best for you, answer a few basic questions:

- What kind of riding will you be doing? Will you be riding in lots of different terrains or sticking to smooth pavement?
- What is your budget? Bicycle costs can vary greatly from entry-level ones that go for a couple of hundred dollars to ones that cost thousands. Remember too that the bike is not your only expense; you'll also need a helmet, gloves, eye protection, and possibly more, depending on the kind of riding you're planning.
- What is your body type? Body shape and size may be a factor in choosing a bike. Someone who has a significant amount of weight to lose needs to consider weight limitations of wheels that come stock on already-built bikes. All bike shops can direct you to a sturdier wheel that is appropriate for heavier riders.

Once you have determined your basic needs, brush up on the fundamentals of the different kinds of bikes before you hit the local bike shop. The chart opposite gives you the information on the four most common fitness bikes.

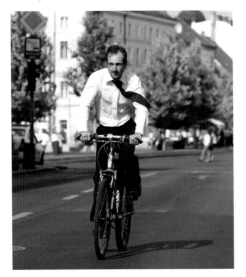

CHOOSE YOUR RIDE

ROAD BIKE

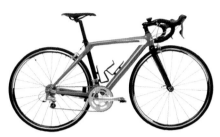

Road bikes are versatile machines that appeal to a wide range of riders, from novices to seasoned cyclists. These lightweight bikes are best on paved roads, and you can use them for pleasure riding, commuting, event rides, touring, and racing. Hybrid models offer you the option of riding off-road on relatively smooth unpaved paths or trails. Basic road bikes usually have a more upright seating position, but many road bikes are also racing bikes, built for speed with low, aerodynamic riding positioning. Accessories include racks, baskets, lighting, and fenders for commuting or touring. Prices range from $300 to $2,000 and upward.

MOUNTAIN BIKE

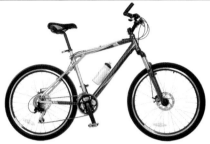

Created for off-road cycling, mountain bikes come with shock-absorbing suspension, large knobby tires, and powerful braking systems, allowing you to tackle just about any terrain, including dirt trails strewn with rocks, roots, and ruts. Their lower gear ratios also help you on steep grades with little or no traction. Although heavier than road bikes, commuters find them appealing, too, because they withstand the stress of potholes. The number of variations is increasing all the time, becoming the choice for cross-country, all-day endurance, Freeride, and downhill biking, along with a variety of competition styles. Prices range from $400 to $2,000 and upward.

CYCLOCROSS BIKE

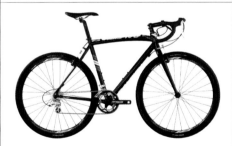

Cyclocross is an increasingly popular sport that involves multiple laps on short courses that feature a variety of terrain, including pavement, dirt, and grass. With its focus on the rider's endurance and bike-handling skills, obstacles are set up so that riders must dismount and carry their bikes around or over them. With a similar design to road bikes meant for racing, cyclocross bikes are lightweight but durable enough to handle extreme conditions. Prices range from $500 to $1,500 and upward.

TRACK BIKE

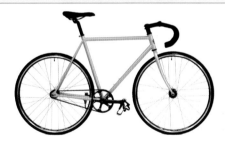

Track bikes are event-specific machines meant for use in a track race within the rules of an indoor or outdoor velodrome. Unlike other bicycles, track bikes feature a fixed-gear system—meaning they have only one gear and no freewheel. They also lack a braking system, which lessens the chance of unpredictable movements during a race. Their narrow tires are inflated to high pressure to reduce rolling resistance. Prices range from $300 to $2,000 and upward.

FULL-BODY ANATOMY

FRONT

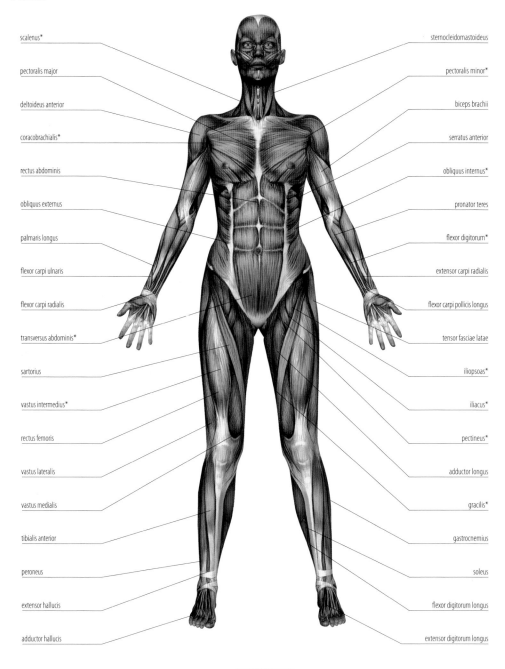

scalenus*

pectoralis major

deltoideus anterior

coracobrachialis*

rectus abdominis

obliquus externus

palmaris longus

flexor carpi ulnaris

flexor carpi radialis

transversus abdominis*

sartorius

vastus intermedius*

rectus femoris

vastus lateralis

vastus medialis

tibialis anterior

peroneus

extensor hallucis

adductor hallucis

sternocleidomastoideus

pectoralis minor*

biceps brachii

serratus anterior

obliquus internus*

pronator teres

flexor digitorum*

extensor carpi radialis

flexor carpi pollicis longus

tensor fasciae latae

iliopsoas*

iliacus*

pectineus*

adductor longus

gracilis*

gastrocnemius

soleus

flexor digitorum longus

extensor digitorum longus

ANNOTATION KEY

* indicates deep muscles

BACK

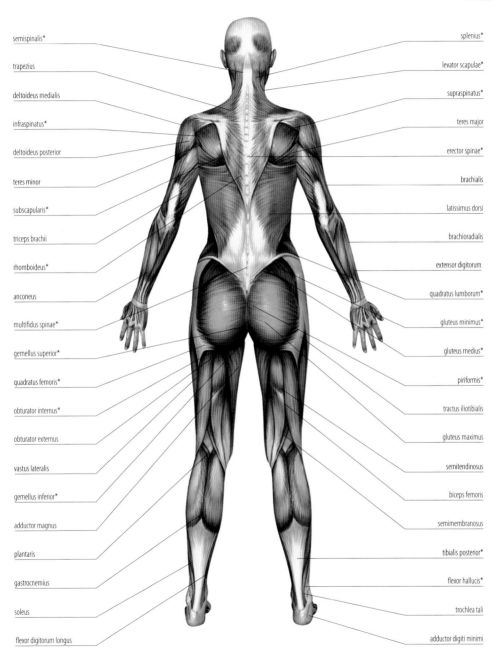

semispinalis*

trapezius

deltoideus medialis

infraspinatus*

deltoideus posterior

teres minor

subscapularis*

triceps brachii

rhomboideus*

anconeus

multifidus spinae*

gemellus superior*

quadratus femoris*

obturator internus*

obturator externus

vastus lateralis

gemellus inferior*

adductor magnus

plantaris

gastrocnemius

soleus

flexor digitorum longus

splenius*

levator scapulae*

supraspinatus*

teres major

erector spinae*

brachialis

latissimus dorsi

brachioradialis

extensor digitorum

quadratus lumborum*

gluteus minimus*

gluteus medius*

piriformis*

tractus iliotibialis

gluteus maximus

semitendinosus

biceps femoris

semimembranosus

tibialis posterior*

flexor hallucis*

trochlea tali

adductor digiti minimi

ANNOTATION KEY

* indicates deep muscles

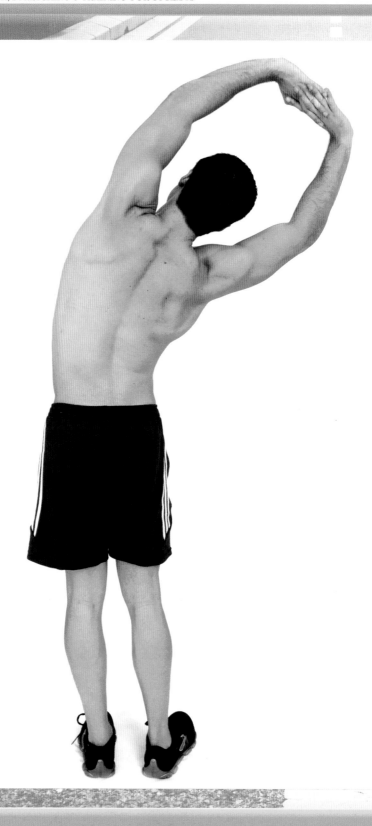

KEEPING FLEXIBLE

M any aspiring and established athletes overlook the importance of flexibility; too often, getting the heart rate up through cardiovascular exercise or powering through a weight-lifting routine takes center stage. Yet flexibility exercises carry immense benefits.

For cyclists, who may spend hours crouching over their handlebars, stretching plays an important role in counteracting the muscles' tightness that can result from performing the repetitive action of pedaling. Stretching consistently—and holding each stretch for 15 seconds—can dramatically increase your range of motion, which in turn helps to decrease the risk of injury as your muscles become more elastic. Stretching also increases blood flow so that more nourishment can reach muscles, and waste products that build up in working muscles, such as lactic acid, can be more effectively removed. The following exercises improve flexibility in your legs as well as your hips, back, abdominals, and glutes, offering a head-to-toe stretch.

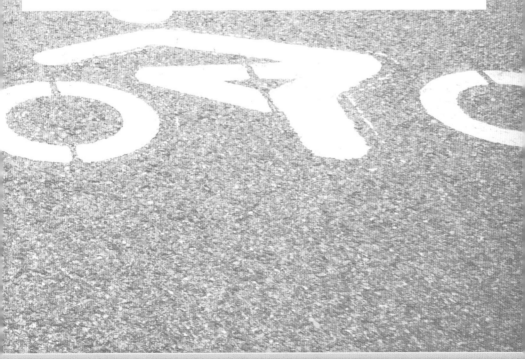

CERVICAL STARS

BEGINNER

THE MUSCLES OF YOUR NECK and upper back do quite a bit of work supporting the weight of your head, making neck pain one of the most common overuse injuries that cyclists suffer. Stretching and strengthening the muscles of your neck is therefore essential. Cervical Stars combines the key actions of flexion, extension, rotation, and lateral rotation to give you a complete neck stretch.

ANNOTATION KEY

Black text indicates strengthening muscles
Gray text indicates stretching muscles
- - - - indicates deep muscles

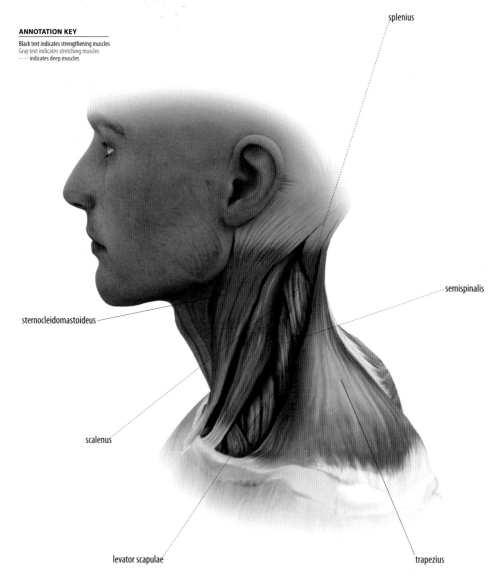

splenius

semispinalis

sternocleidomastoideus

scalenus

levator scapulae

trapezius

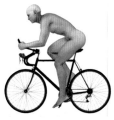

HOW TO DO IT

1 Sit or stand, keeping your neck, shoulders, and torso straight. Keeping your chin level, look straight ahead.

2 Imagine that there is a star in front of you with a vertical line, a horizontal line, and two diagonal lines. Trace the star shape with your head and neck by following the vertical line up and down three times.

3 Next, follow the horizontal line once.

4 Finally, trace the two diagonal lines.

5 Return to the starting position, and repeat five times.

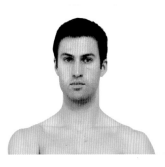

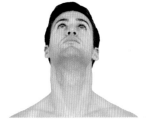

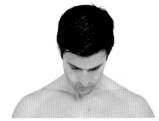

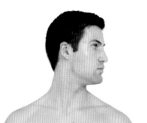

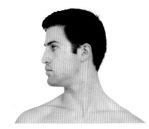

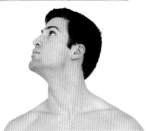

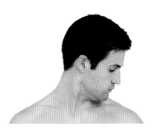

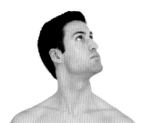

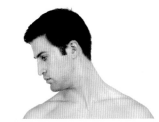

PRIMARY TARGETS
- splenius
- sternocleidomastoideus
- levator scapulae
- scalenus
- semispinalis
- trapezius

BENEFITS
- Improves range of motion
- Stretches neck rotators, flexors, extensors, and lateral flexors
- Relieves neck pain

CAUTIONS
- Numbness running down your arm or into your hand

PERFECT YOUR FORM
- Move smoothly and with control.
- Avoid hunching or tensing your shoulders.

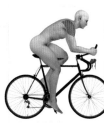

SHOULDER STRETCH

BENDING FORWARD while looking up isn't a natural human position, which is why so many cyclists feel tension in their neck and shoulders after a long ride. To counteract the effects of the forward-flexed position, be sure to perform flexibility exercises, such as the Shoulder Stretch, to relieve any tightness and tension.

PRIMARY TARGETS
- deltoideus posterior
- triceps brachii
- obliquus externus
- teres minor
- infraspinatus

BENEFITS
- Stretches shoulders, preventing stiffness

CAUTIONS
- Shoulder injury

PERFECT YOUR FORM
- Keep your elbow straight while you apply pressure with your hand.
- Avoid allowing your shoulders to lift toward your ears.

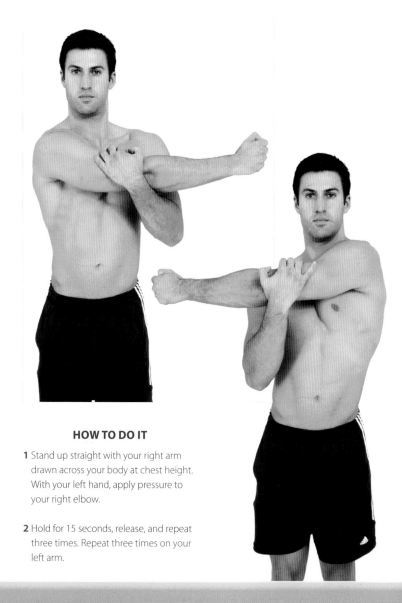

HOW TO DO IT

1 Stand up straight with your right arm drawn across your body at chest height. With your left hand, apply pressure to your right elbow.

2 Hold for 15 seconds, release, and repeat three times. Repeat three times on your left arm.

TRAPEZIUS STRETCH

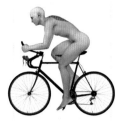

THE TRAPEZIUS MUSCLE runs along the sides of the neck and shoulders, attaching at the base of the head. Cyclists tend to tense these muscles while riding, decreasing blood flow to the area—which can lead to pain and muscle spasms. Stretch this area regularly to keep your neck strong, limber, and pain-free.

PRIMARY TARGETS
- scalenus
- sternocleidomastoideus
- trapezius

BENEFITS
- Stretches upper back and neck

CAUTIONS
- Shoulder injury

PERFECT YOUR FORM
- Keep the shoulder of your resting arm pressed down, away from your ear.
- Avoid twisting your torso.

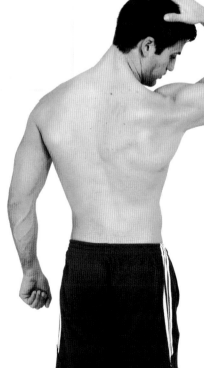

HOW TO DO IT

1 Standing with your feet parallel and shoulder-width apart, gently grasp the side of your head with your right hand.

2 Tilt your head toward your raised elbow until you feel the stretch in the side of your neck.

3 Turn your head toward your right shoulder as you continue to feel the stretch.

4 Hold for 15 seconds, and repeat. Switch sides, and repeat the sequence on the left side.

CHEST STRETCH

BEGINNER

THE CHEST STRETCH will help counteract the effects of long hours spent in the forward-leaning position of cycling. It offers a backward stretch to the pectoral muscles of your chest and the deltoids of your shoulders.

ANNOTATION KEY

Black text indicates strengthening muscles
Gray text indicates stretching muscles
- - - - indicates deep muscles

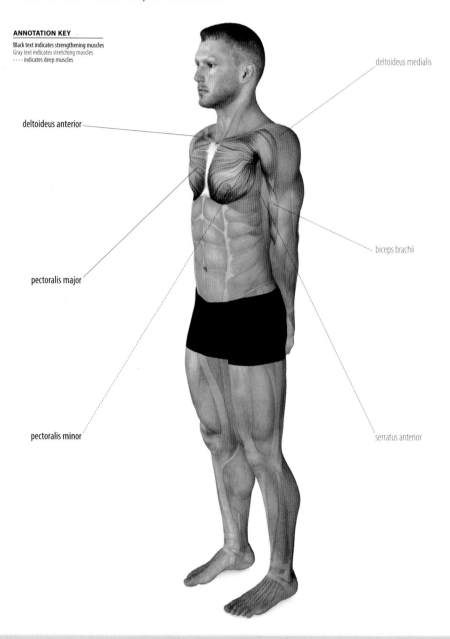

deltoideus medialis

deltoideus anterior

pectoralis major

biceps brachii

pectoralis minor

serratus anterior

HOW TO DO IT

1 Stand straight with your arms behind your back and your hands clasped together.

2 Pinch your shoulder blades together as you reach and lift your arms away from your body, making sure to keep your elbows straight.

3 Hold for 15 seconds before returning your arms to the starting position. Repeat.

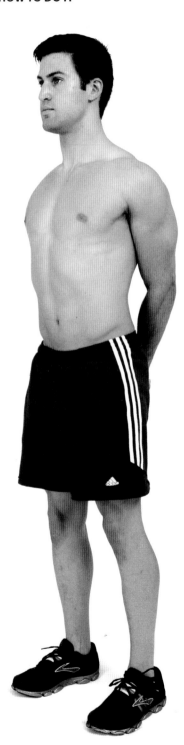

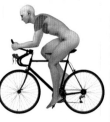

PRIMARY TARGETS
- pectoralis major
- pectoralis minor
- deltoideus anterior
- biceps brachii

BENEFITS
- Stretches pectoral muscles and fronts of shoulders

CAUTIONS
- Shoulder injury

PERFECT YOUR FORM
- Press your shoulders down, away from your ears.
- Elongate your arms and shoulders as much as possible.
- Avoid hunching your shoulders.
- Avoid twisting your neck.

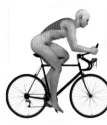

LOWER & UPPER BACK STRETCH

The LOWER & UPPER BACK STRETCH will help gets the kinks out of a tight back, while also giving your hamstrings a stretch.

PRIMARY TARGETS
- supraspinatus
- infraspinatus
- teres minor
- subscapularis
- teres major
- latissimus dorsi
- erector spinae
- quadratus lumborum
- multifidus spinae

BENEFITS
- Stretches back and hamstrings

CAUTIONS
- Lower-back pain
- Neck injury

PERFECT YOUR FORM
- Keep your legs extended and on the floor.
- Keep your forearms resting slightly above your knees.
- Avoid leaning too far, too quickly; instead, stretch gradually.

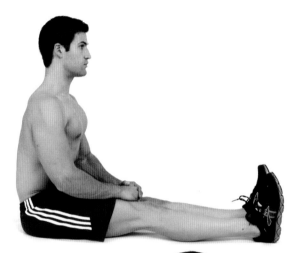

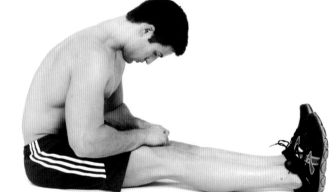

HOW TO DO IT

1 Sit on the floor with your legs extended in front of you, your ankles bent at a 90-degree angle so that your toes point toward the ceiling.

2 Loosely clasp your hands, and rest your forearms on your knees, bending your torso forward from your hips.

3 Without bouncing, continue to lean forward, concentrating on stretching your entire spine.

4 Hold at your lowest point for about 15 seconds, and repeat.

SCOOP RHOMBOIDS

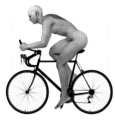

YOUR RHOMBOIDS ARE A LAYER of deep muscles that keep your shoulder blades pressed against your thoracic spine for stability. They work in concert with your trapezius and other shoulder muscles to retract and protract your shoulders. The Scoop Rhomboids stretch will help maintain easy back mobility.

PRIMARY TARGETS
• rhomboideus

BENEFITS
• Stretches upper back
• Improves mobility in back muscles
• Reduces tension

CAUTIONS
• Lower-back pain

PERFECT YOUR FORM
• Keep your breath steady, focusing on exhalation as you round your upper back and lean backward.
• Avoid holding your breath.

HOW TO DO IT

1 Sit on the floor and extend your legs in front of you in a parallel position. Bend your knees slightly, keeping your heels on the floor.

2 Grasp beneath your hamstrings with your hands.

3 Keeping your chin down, round your upper back down as you lean back toward the floor. Hold this position for 10 to 15 seconds.

4 Slowly roll up to the starting position, and repeat if desired.

LATISSIMUS DORSI STRETCH

BEGINNER

THE LATISSIMUS DORSI is a broad muscle stretching from the back of your shoulder to the center of your spine. Stretching this muscle can help ease the tension of sitting in the forward-leaning position of cycling.

ANNOTATION KEY

Black text indicates strengthening muscles
Gray text indicates stretching muscles
---- indicates deep muscles

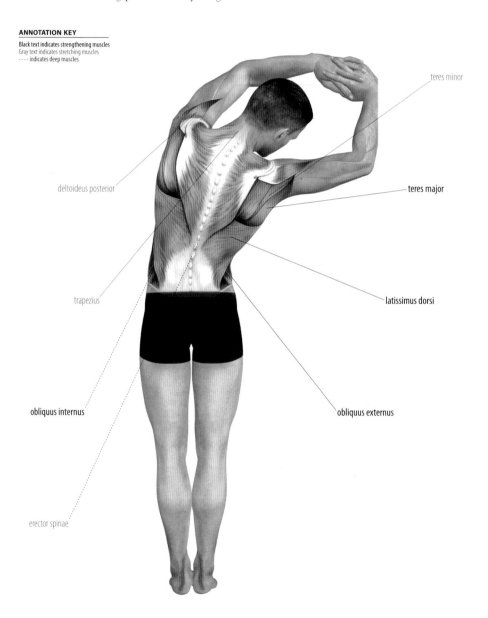

teres minor

deltoideus posterior

teres major

trapezius

latissimus dorsi

obliquus internus

obliquus externus

erector spinae

HOW TO DO IT

1 Clasp your hands together above your head, your palms turned upward toward the ceiling.

2 Reach your hands outward as you make a circular pattern with your torso.

3 Slowly make a full circle. Repeat sequence three times in each direction.

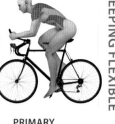

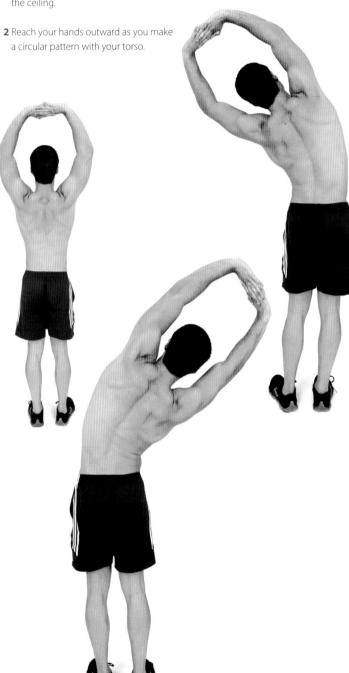

PRIMARY TARGETS
- latissimus dorsi
- obliquus internus

BENEFITS
- Stretches back, obliques, and shoulders

CAUTIONS
- Shoulder injury

PERFECT YOUR FORM
- Avoid leaning back as you come to the top of the circle.

SPINAL TWIST

BEGINNER

To counteract any back stiffness you might experience after a long ride, perform exercises that offer a rotational stretch. Spinal Twist will help increase the range of motion in your upper body, stretching the muscles of your back and torso while strongly maintaining a central vertical axis through your body.

ANNOTATION KEY

Black text indicates strengthening muscles
Gray text indicates stretching muscles
- - - - indicates deep muscles

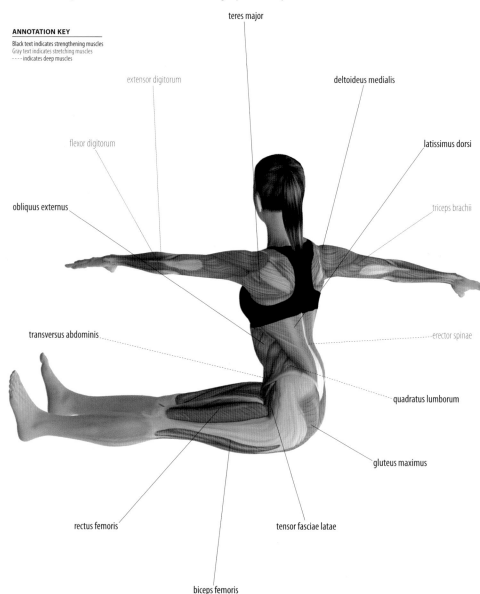

teres major

extensor digitorum

deltoideus medialis

flexor digitorum

latissimus dorsi

obliquus externus

triceps brachii

transversus abdominis

erector spinae

quadratus lumborum

gluteus maximus

rectus femoris

tensor fasciae latae

biceps femoris

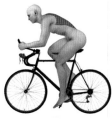

HOW TO DO IT

1 Sit on the floor with your back straight. Extend your legs in front of you slightly more than hip-width apart.

2 Lift yourself as tall as you can from the base of your spine. Ground your hips into the floor.

3 Lift up and out of your hips as you pull in your lower abdominals. Twist from your waist to the left, keeping your hips squared and grounded.

4 Slowly return to the center.

5 Lift up and out of your hips again, twisting in the other direction.

6 Return to the center. Repeat three times in each direction.

PRIMARY TARGETS
- erector spinae
- obliquus externus
- transversus abdominis
- biceps femoris
- gluteus maximus
- tensor fasciae latae
- latissimus dorsi
- teres major
- quadratus lumborum
- deltoideus medialis
- rectus femoris

BENEFITS
- Stretches spinal muscles
- Strengthens and lengthens torso

CAUTIONS
- Back pain

PERFECT YOUR FORM
- If your hamstrings are too tight to allow you to sit up straight, place a towel under your buttocks, and bend your knees slightly.
- Rotate your torso along the central axis of your body.
- Keep your arms parallel to the floor.
- Avoid allowing your hips to rise off the floor.

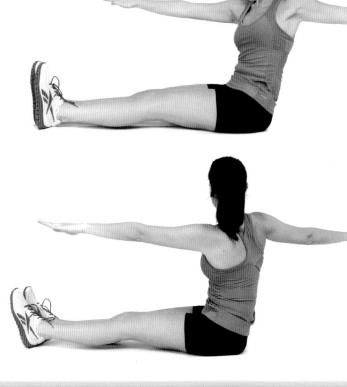

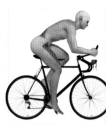

SPINE STRETCH

THE SPINE STRETCH works to increase the length and flexibility of your spine, which is essential to good posture. It also gives your lower back, hips, and thighs a beneficial stretch.

PRIMARY TARGETS
• erector spinae
• quadratus lumborum
• vastus lateralis
• tractus iliotibialis
• tensor fasciae latae

BENEFITS
• Stretches lower back, hips, and thighs

CAUTIONS
• Hip injury
• Lower-back injury

PERFECT YOUR FORM
• Relax your lower back.
• Avoid allowing your shoulders to lift off the floor.

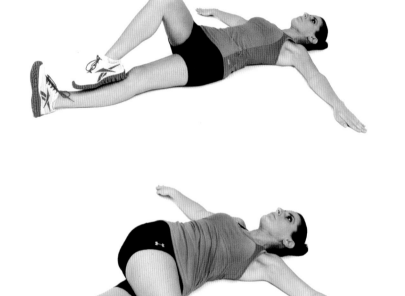

HOW TO DO IT

1 Lie on your back with your legs extended. Keeping your left leg straight, bend your right leg and place your right foot on your left shin.

2 Keeping both shoulders on the floor, bring your right leg across your body

until you feel the stretch in the area between your lower back and hips. Stretch only as far as your can while keeping your shoulders on the floor.

3 Hold for 15 seconds, and repeat sequence three times on each side.

LUMBAR STRETCH

THE LUMBAR STRETCH is another stretch that works your spine, with a particular emphasis on the lower back. Performing this stretch will open up your back and increase its flexibility. Try to get your knees as close to the floor as possible, but not past the point of pain.

PRIMARY TARGETS
- quadratus lumborum
- erector spinae
- obliquus externus

BENEFITS
- Stretches lower back, hips, thighs, and oblique muscles

CAUTIONS
- Lower-back pain
- Hip injury

PERFECT YOUR FORM
- Relax your lower back.
- Avoid allowing your shoulders to lift off the floor.

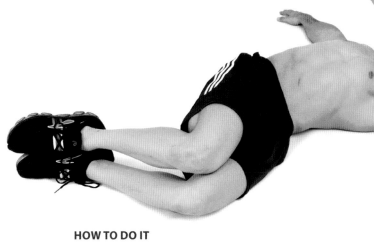

HOW TO DO IT

1 Lie flat on the floor with both feet and knees together, your knees bent.

2 Slowly rock your knees from side to side until you feel a stretch along your lower back through the hips or until your knees reach the floor. Repeat 10 times.

COBRA STRETCH

BEGINNER

The Cobra Stretch takes its inspiration from the yoga pose that resembles the raised-hood stance of a cobra about to strike. When you properly execute this stretch, your body will take on the raised-hood position. It slowly stretches your entire spinal column and the muscles surrounding it, as well as stretches your glutes, chest, and abdominals.

ANNOTATION KEY
Black text indicates strengthening muscles
Gray text indicates stretching muscles
---- indicates deep muscles

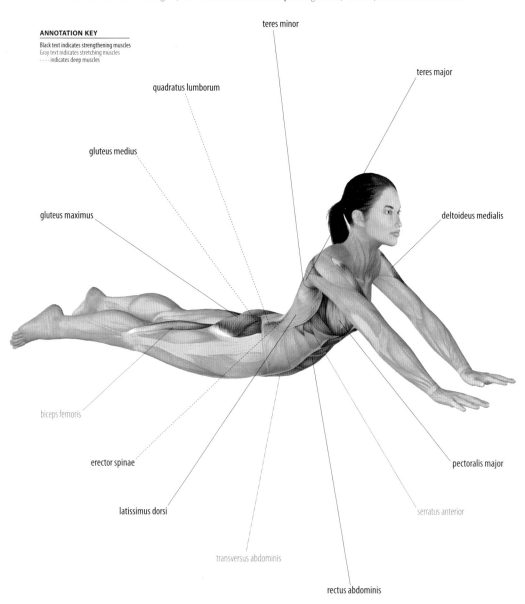

teres minor

teres major

quadratus lumborum

gluteus medius

gluteus maximus

deltoideus medialis

biceps femoris

erector spinae

pectoralis major

latissimus dorsi

serratus anterior

transversus abdominis

rectus abdominis

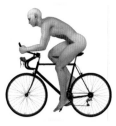

HOW TO DO IT

1 Lie prone on the floor. Bend your elbows, placing your hands flat on the floor beside your chest. Keep your elbows pulled in toward your body. Extend your legs, pressing your pubis, thighs, and tops of your feet into the floor.

2 Push down into the floor, and slowly lift through the top of your chest as you straighten your arms.

3 Pull your tailbone down toward your pubis as you push your shoulders down and back.

4 Elongate your neck and gaze forward.

5 Hold for up to 15 to 30 seconds, and exhale as you lower yourself to the floor.

PRIMARY TARGETS
- quadratus lumborum
- erector spinae
- latissimus dorsi
- gluteus maximus
- gluteus medius
- pectoralis major
- rectus abdominis
- deltoideus medialis
- teres major
- teres minor

BENEFITS
- Strengthens spine and buttocks
- Stretches chest, abdominals, and shoulders

CAUTIONS
- Back injury

PERFECT YOUR FORM
- Lift out of your chest and back, rather than depending too much on your arms to create the arch in your back.
- Keep your shoulders and elbows pressed back to create more lift in your chest.
- Don't tense your buttocks, which adds pressure on your lower back.
- Avoid lifting your hips off the floor.

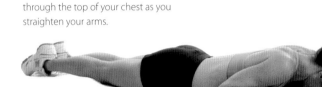

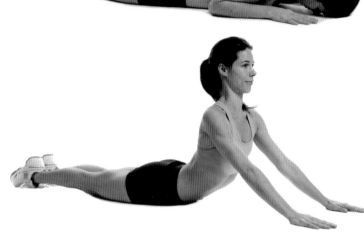

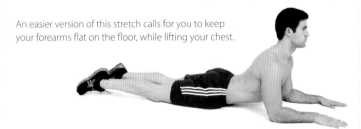

An easier version of this stretch calls for you to keep your forearms flat on the floor, while lifting your chest.

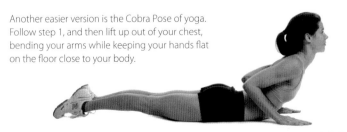

Another easier version is the Cobra Pose of yoga. Follow step 1, and then lift up out of your chest, bending your arms while keeping your hands flat on the floor close to your body.

SUPINE FIGURE 4

BEGINNER

THE PIRIFORMIS IS A SMALL pear-shaped muscle, lying deep behind the gluteals, which rotates your hips. If your piriformis muscles becomes too tight, they can impinge on your sciatic nerve, resulting in pain radiating from your buttocks, down your thigh, and up into your spine. The Supine Figure 4 targets this important muscle, so lie flat on a mat, distributing your weight evenly, to obtain an effective, controlled stretch.

ANNOTATION KEY

Black text indicates strengthening muscles
Gray text indicates stretching muscles
- - - - indicates deep muscles

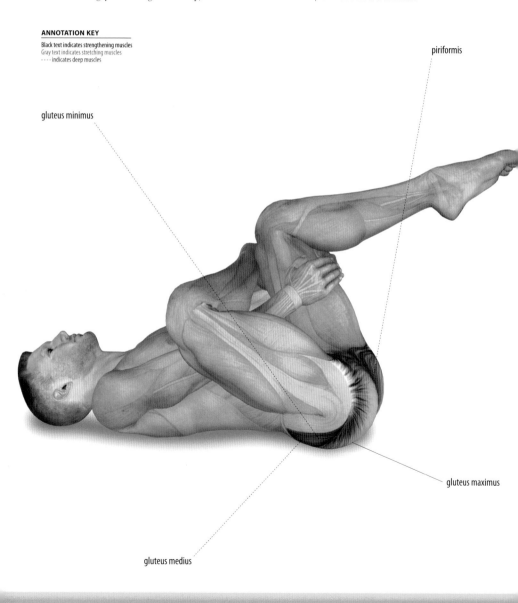

piriformis

gluteus minimus

gluteus maximus

gluteus medius

HOW TO DO IT

1 Lie on your back with your legs extended and toes pointed.

2 Bend your right knee and turn your leg out so that your right ankle rests on your left thigh just above the knee, creating a the shape of a figure 4.

3 Bend your left leg, drawing both legs (still in the figure 4 position) in toward your chest as you grasp the back of your left thigh.

4 Push your right elbow against your right inner thigh, slightly turning out your right leg to increase the intensity of the stretch.

5 Return to the starting position, switch legs, and repeat.

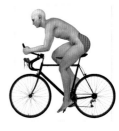

PRIMARY TARGETS
• gluteus maximus
• gluteus medius
• gluteus minimus
• piriformis

BENEFITS
• Stretches glutes and lower back

CAUTIONS
• Knee issues
• Severe lower-back pain

PERFECT YOUR FORM
• Keep your head and shoulder blades on the floor.
• Relax your hips so that you can go deeper into the stretch.
• Perform the stretch slowly.

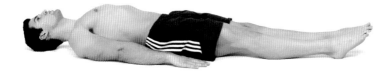

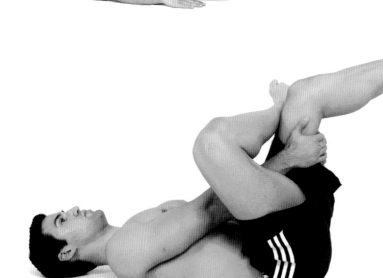

BUTTERFLY STRETCH

INTERMEDIATE

THE BUTTERFLY STRETCH is a yoga-inspired stretch. It targets the all-important hip adductor muscles of your inner thighs, as well as other muscles of the groin, hips, and lower back that flex, straighten, rotate, and adduct your hip joint.

ANNOTATION KEY

Black text indicates strengthening muscles
Gray text indicates stretching muscles
- - - - indicates deep muscles

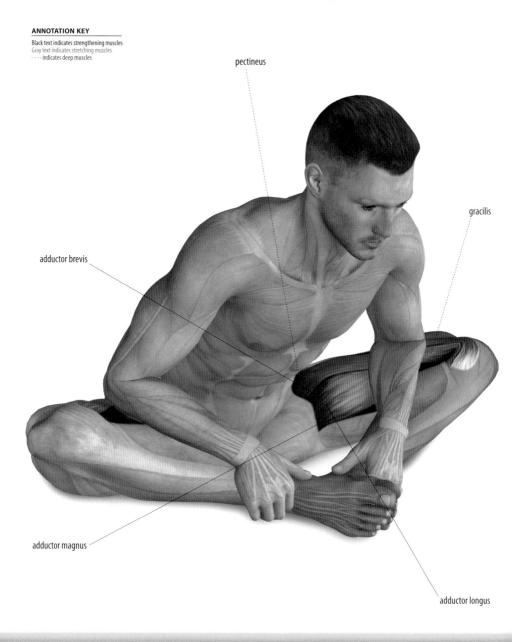

pectineus

gracilis

adductor brevis

adductor magnus

adductor longus

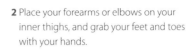

HOW TO DO IT

1 Sit up tall on the floor or a mat with the soles of your feet pressed together.

2 Place your forearms or elbows on your inner thighs, and grab your feet and toes with your hands.

3 Draw your heels in toward your core.

4 Fold your upper body forward until you feel a stretch in your groin and in your upper inner thighs.

5 Slowly roll up, and repeat if desired.

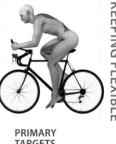

PRIMARY TARGETS
• adductor longus
• adductor magnus
• adductor brevis
• gracilis
• pectineus
• obturator externus
• erector spinae
• quadratus lumborum

BENEFITS
• Stretches hips and lower back
• Prevents and counteracts soreness caused by long bike rides

CAUTIONS
• Hip issues
• Lower-back issues

PERFECT YOUR FORM
• Avoid slouching.
• Don't hold your breath.
• Avoid rocking backward, off your hip bones; instead, feel them anchored on the floor.
• Exhale as you drop your chest toward the floor.

HIP ADDUCTOR STRETCH

BEGINNER

EXERCISES THAT COUNTERBALANCE the repeated flexion and extension of pedaling a bike are essential components of a cyclist's workout. The Hip Adductor Stretch targets the inner thigh muscles, including the pectineus, along with the hamstrings and piriformis.

ANNOTATION KEY

Black text indicates strengthening muscles
Gray text indicates stretching muscles
- - - - indicates deep muscles

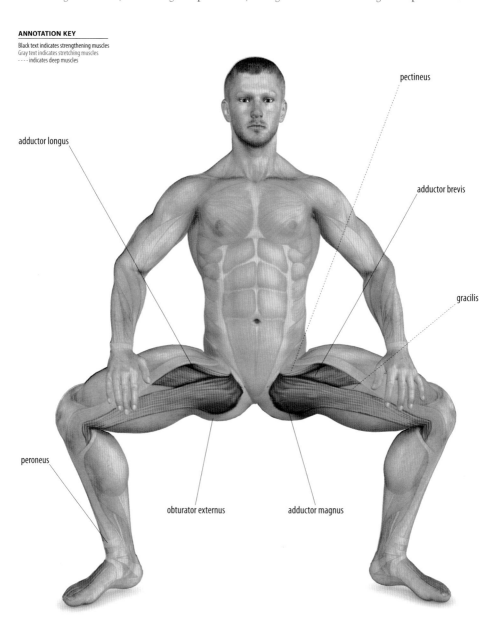

pectineus

adductor longus

adductor brevis

gracilis

peroneus

obturator externus

adductor magnus

HOW TO DO IT

1 Standing, separate your feet wider than hip width, so that you are in a straddle position. Bend your knees.

2 Place your hands on your knees and bend at your hips, keeping your spine in a neutral position and your shoulders slightly forward.

3 Keeping your torso in the same position and your hips behind your heels, shift your weight to one side, bending your knee while extending your opposite leg. Hold for 10 seconds, and repeat on the other side.

KEEPING FLEXIBLE

PRIMARY TARGETS
- adductor longus
- adductor magnus
- peroneus
- biceps femoris
- semitendinosus
- semimembranosus
- piriformis

BENEFITS
- Stretches hips, hamstrings, and gluteal muscles

CAUTIONS
- Hip injury
- Knee injury

PERFECT YOUR FORM
- Keep your trunk aligned as you move from side to side.
- Place your hand on your thighs to assist your posture.
- Relax your neck and shoulders.
- Avoid rounding your spine.
- Avoid allowing your feet to shift or lift off the floor.
- Avoid allowing your knees to extend over your toes while bending.

HIP FLEXOR STRETCH

BEGINNER

HIP FLEXIBILITY IS A MUST FOR CYCLISTS, but the repeated flexion of pedaling can result in tightness from overuse. Regularly perform the Hip Flexor Stretch to ensure that your hips stay supple and limber while also stretching the hamstring muscles of your thigh.

ANNOTATION KEY

Black text indicates strengthening muscles
Gray text indicates stretching muscles
- - - - indicates deep muscles

pectineus

obliquus externus

iliopsoas

adductor magnus

gracilis

vastus medialis

semitendinosus

adductor longus

biceps femoris

tensor fasciae latae

semimembranosus

vastus intermedius

rectus femoris

vastus lateralis

HOW TO DO IT

1 Kneeling, bring one leg forward with your foot in front of your knee.

2 Slowly lean forward and push your pelvis downward until you feel a stretch in the front of your hip. Hold for 15 seconds. Switch legs, and repeat, completing the sequence three times on each leg.

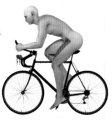

PRIMARY TARGETS
- rectus femoris
- vastus medialis
- biceps femoris
- tensor fasciae latae

BENEFITS
- Stretches hamstrings and hip flexors

CAUTIONS
- Hip injury
- Knee injury

PERFECT YOUR FORM
- Face forward and keep your back straight.
- Avoid pushing your front knee past your ankle. The angle that your calf forms with the mat should not exceed 90 degrees.

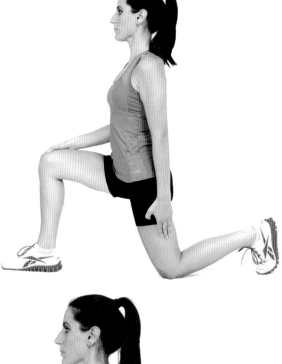

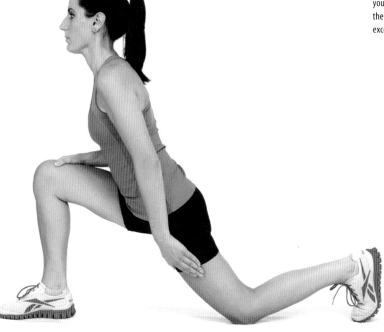

HIP/ILIOTIBIAL BAND STRETCH

INTERMEDIATE

KEEP YOUR HIPS FLEXIBLE and your iliotibial bands supple to counteract the effects of
the repetitive motions of cycling. Use the Hip/Iliotibial Band Stretch to stretch these
areas while also providing yourself with a full spinal and abdominal twist.

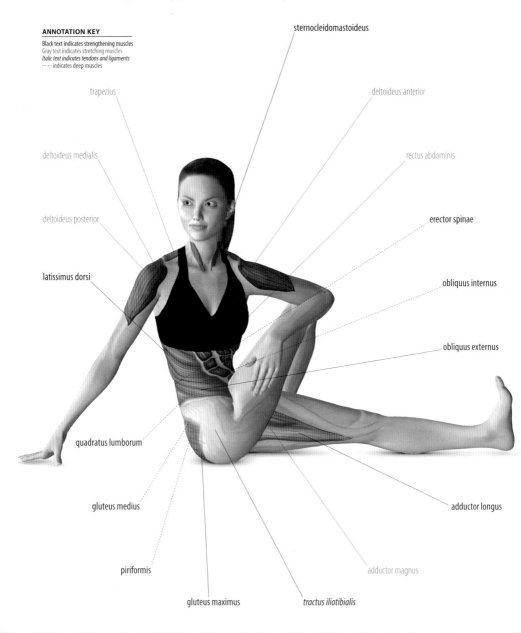

ANNOTATION KEY
Black text indicates strengthening muscles
Gray text indicates stretching muscles
Italic text indicates tendons and ligaments
---- indicates deep muscles

sternocleidomastoideus

trapezius

deltoideus anterior

deltoideus medialis

rectus abdominis

deltoideus posterior

erector spinae

latissimus dorsi

obliquus internus

obliquus externus

quadratus lumborum

gluteus medius

adductor longus

piriformis

adductor magnus

gluteus maximus

tractus iliotibialis

HOW TO DO IT

1 Sit on the floor, sitting up as straight as possible with your back flattened and your legs extended in front of you in a parallel position. Your feet should be relaxed and flexed slightly.

2 Extend your left leg straight in front of you, and bend your right knee. Cross your bent knee over the straight leg, and keep your foot flat on the floor.

3 Wrap your left arm around the bent knee so that you are able to apply pressure to your leg to rotate your torso.

4 Keeping your hips aligned, rotate your upper spine as you pull your chest in toward your knee.

5 Hold for 30 seconds. Slowly release, and repeat three times on each side.

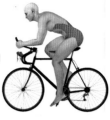

PRIMARY TARGETS
- adductor longus
- iliopsoas
- rhomboideus
- sternocleidomastoideus
- latissimus dorsi
- obliquus internus
- obliquus externus
- quadratus lumborum
- erector spinae
- multifidus spinae
- tractus iliotibialis
- gluteus maximus
- gluteus medius
- piriformis

BENEFITS
- Stretches hip extensors and flexors
- Stretches obliques

CAUTIONS
- Severe lower-back pain

PERFECT YOUR FORM
- Apply even pressure to your leg with your active hand.
- Keep your torso upright as you pull your knee and torso together.
- Avoid lifting the foot of your bent leg off the floor.

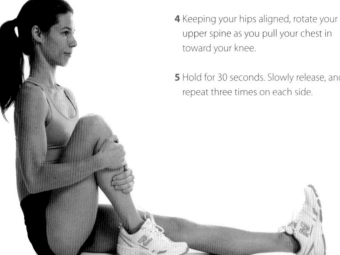

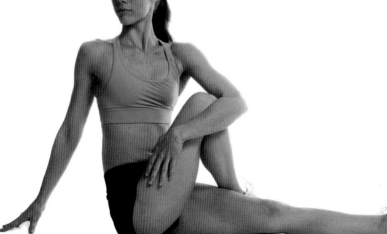

ILIOTIBIAL BAND STRETCH

BEGINNER

THE ILIOTIBIAL BAND is a thick band of connective tissue that crosses your hip joint and extends down to insert on your kneecap, tibia, and biceps femoris tendon. The iliotibial band stabilizes your knee and abducts your hip. Perform the Iliotibial Band Stretch as a pre-cycle stretch and before attempting any of the more demanding lower-body exercises included in this book.

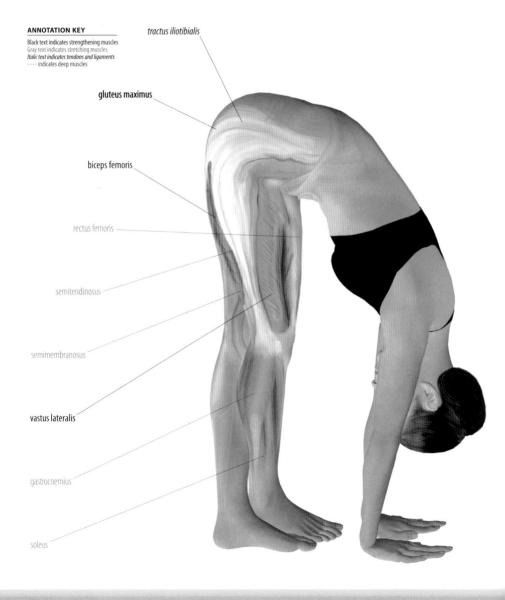

ANNOTATION KEY

Black text indicates strengthening muscles
Gray text indicates stretching muscles
Italic text indicates tendons and ligaments
- - - - indicates deep muscles

tractus iliotibialis

gluteus maximus

biceps femoris

rectus femoris

semitendinosus

semimembranosus

vastus lateralis

gastrocnemius

soleus

HOW TO DO IT

1 Standing, cross your left leg in front of your right.

2 Bend forward from the hips while keeping both legs straight, and reach your hands toward the floor.

3 Hold for 15 seconds. Repeat the sequence three times on each leg.

If you are not yet flexible enough to place your palms flat on the floor, just aim to lightly touch your fingertips to the floor while keeping both feet firmly planted.

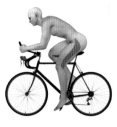

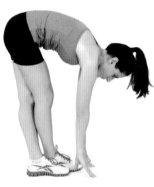

PRIMARY TARGETS
- tractus iliotibialis
- biceps femoris
- gluteus maximus
- vastus lateralis

BENEFITS
- Helps to stabilize knee joints
- Helps to keep hips flexible
- Stretches back, hamstrings, and calves

CAUTIONS
- Neck issues
- Lower-back pain

PERFECT YOUR FORM
- Stretch with good alignment so that your back leg and your spine form a straight line.
- Avoid lifting your back heel off the floor.
- Avoid arching or rounding your back.
- Avoid forcing your hands to reach the floor.

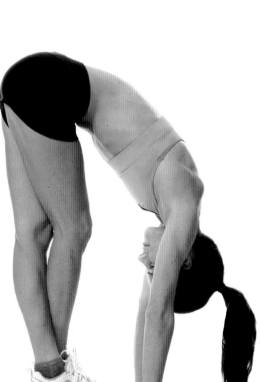

FORWARD LUNGE

BEGINNER

THE FORWARD LUNGE is an excellent stretching exercise that targets your glutes and your quadriceps, along with your hamstrings and hip flexor muscles. Keeping them in top condition will allow you to cycle with power and control for longer stretches of time.

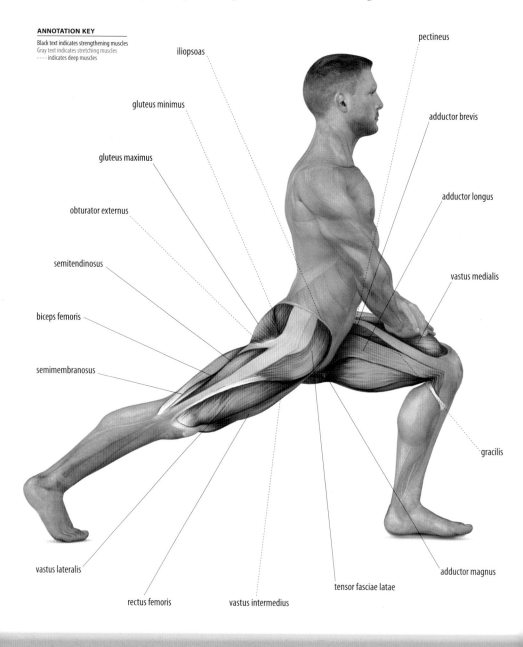

ANNOTATION KEY

Black text indicates strengthening muscles
Gray text indicates stretching muscles
---- indicates deep muscles

iliopsoas

pectineus

gluteus minimus

adductor brevis

gluteus maximus

obturator externus

adductor longus

semitendinosus

vastus medialis

biceps femoris

semimembranosus

gracilis

vastus lateralis

adductor magnus

rectus femoris

vastus intermedius

tensor fasciae latae

HOW TO DO IT

1 Stand with your legs and feet parallel and shoulder-width apart, and your knees bent very slightly. Tuck your pelvis slightly forward, lift your chest, and press your shoulders down and back.

2 Bend your left knee, and step your right leg back behind your body, extending it straight.

3 Place your palms on your knee, and hold for 15 seconds.

4 Release the stretch, switch legs and repeat on the other side.

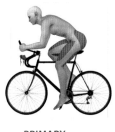

PRIMARY TARGETS
- rectus femoris
- vastus lateralis
- vastus intermedius
- vastus medialis
- biceps femoris
- semitendinosus
- semimembranosus
- gluteus maximus
- adductor longus
- adductor magnus
- adductor brevis
- iliopsoas
- gracilis
- pectineus
- tensor fasciae latae
- obturator externus
- gluteus minimus

BENEFITS
- Stretches hip flexors
- Strengthens hamstrings, thighs, and glutes

CAUTIONS
- Severe hip or knee degeneration

PERFECT YOUR FORM
- Keep your back leg extended in line with your hips to form one long straight line.
- Keep your knee directly above your ankle.
- Avoid dropping your back extended leg to the floor.
- Avoid hunching your shoulders.

STANDING QUADS STRETCH

BEGINNER

THE QUADRICEPS FEMORIS GROUP is the long muscles that sit on the front aspect of your thigh. It is essential for you to stretch this major group of muscles in order to achieve full length and flexibility in your legs. During this stretch, be sure to stand tall, without leaning or rocking, to improve your balance as well.

ANNOTATION KEY

Black text indicates strengthening muscles
Gray text indicates stretching muscles
- - - - indicates deep muscles

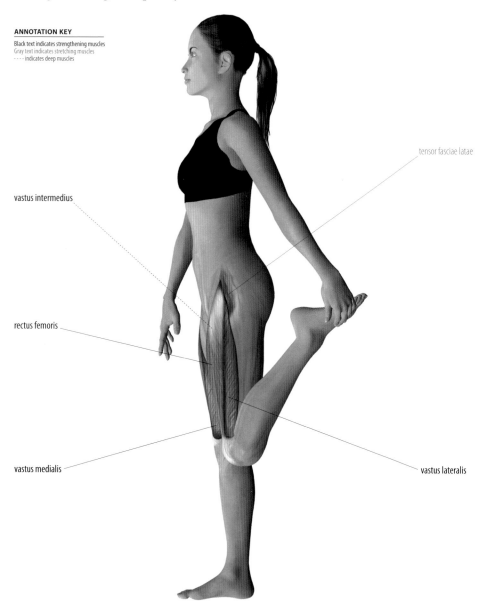

tensor fasciae latae

vastus intermedius

rectus femoris

vastus medialis

vastus lateralis

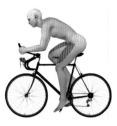

HOW TO DO IT

1 Stand with your feet together. Bend your left leg behind you, and grasp your foot with your left hand. Pull your heel toward your buttocks until you feel a stretch in the front of your thigh. Keep both knees together and aligned.

2 Hold for 15 seconds. Repeat sequence three times on each leg.

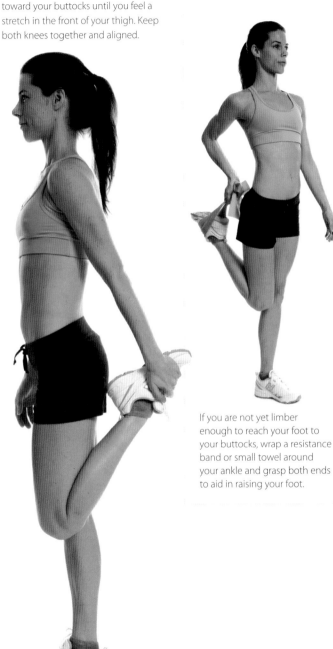

If you are not yet limber enough to reach your foot to your buttocks, wrap a resistance band or small towel around your ankle and grasp both ends to aid in raising your foot.

PRIMARY TARGETS
- rectus femoris
- vastus lateralis
- vastus medialis
- vastus intermedius

BENEFITS
- Helps to keep thigh muscles flexible

CAUTIONS
- Knee issues

PERFECT YOUR FORM
- Both knees to remain pressed together.
- With your arm opposite the bent leg, lean against a wall or other stable object to aid your balance.
- Avoid leaning forward with your chest.
- Avoid bringing your foot closer to your buttocks than you can reach with a comfortable, pain-free stretch—this can compress the knee joint.

SIDE-LYING KNEE BEND

BEGINNER

LIKE THE STANDING QUADS STRETCH, the Side-Lying Knee Bend targets the quadriceps
at the front of your thigh—the rectus femoris, vastus intermedius, vastus lateralis, and
vastus medialis. Cycling strengthens these muscles, but can also tighten them, so be sure
to stretch them regularly to keep them limber and flexible.

ANNOTATION KEY

Black text indicates strengthening muscles
Gray text indicates stretching muscles
- - - - indicates deep muscles

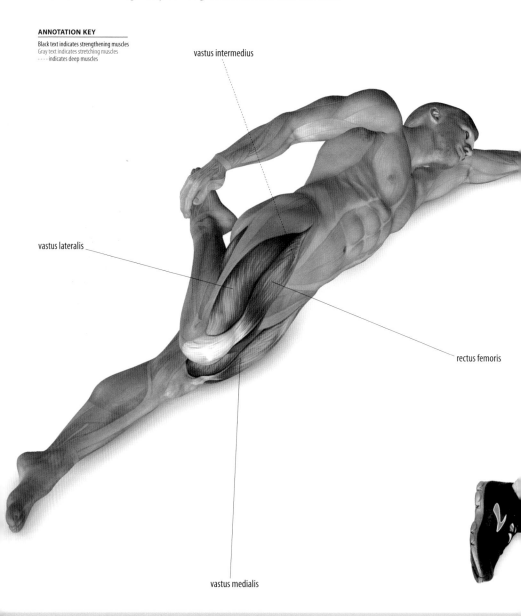

vastus intermedius

vastus lateralis

rectus femoris

vastus medialis

HOW TO DO IT

1 Lie on your left side with your legs extended together in line with your body. Extend your left arm, and rest your head on your upper arm.

2 Bend your right knee and grasp your ankle with your right hand.

3 Pull your ankle in toward your buttocks as you stretch.

4 Return to the starting position, and repeat on the other side.

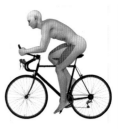

PRIMARY TARGETS
• rectus femoris
• vastus lateralis
• vastus intermedius
• vastus medialis

BENEFITS
• Helps to keep thigh muscles flexible

CAUTIONS
• Knee issues

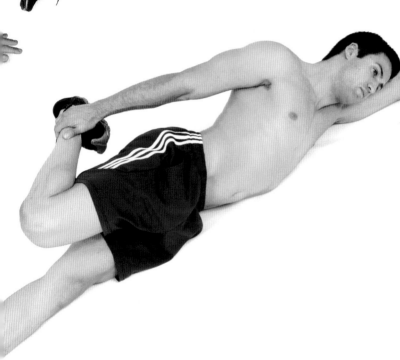

PERFECT YOUR FORM
• Keep your knees together, one on top of the other.
• Tuck your pelvis slightly forward, and lift your chest to engage and stretch your core.
• Keep your foot pointed and parallel with your leg.
• Avoid leaning back onto your glutes.
• Place a towel under your bottom hip if it feels uncomfortable to rest directly on the floor.

UNILATERAL LEG RAISE

INTERMEDIATE

THIS SIMPLE BUT EFFECTIVE STRETCH is important in preparing your lower back, hip extensors, and hip rotators for many of the more intensive exercises in this book. Take care not to overexert your hamstrings. Slow, deliberate stretching is best.

ANNOTATION KEY

Black text indicates strengthening muscles
Gray text indicates stretching muscles
- - - - indicates deep muscles

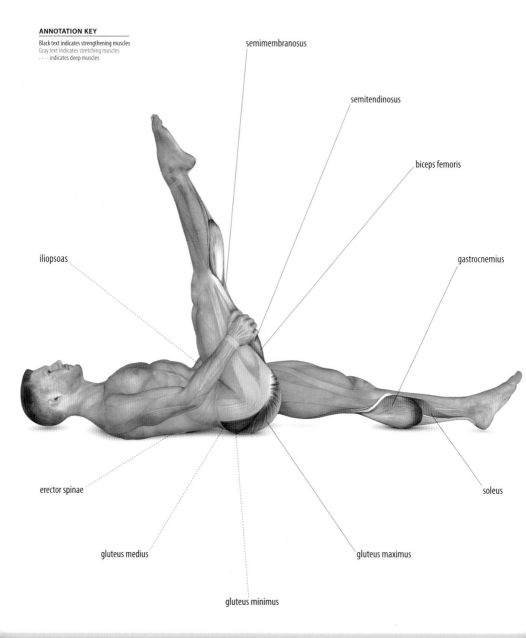

semimembranosus

semitendinosus

biceps femoris

iliopsoas

gastrocnemius

erector spinae

soleus

gluteus medius

gluteus maximus

gluteus minimus

HOW TO DO IT

1 Lie on your back with both legs extended and your spine in a imprinted position so that your lower back touches the floor.

2 With your hands placed on your hamstrings just below the knee, extend and straighten your left leg upward.

3 Point both feet, and hold this position for 15 to 30 seconds.

4 Switch legs, and repeat the stretch on the other side.

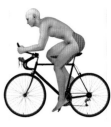

PRIMARY TARGETS

• biceps femoris
• semitendinosus
• semimembranosus
• erector spinae
• gluteus maximus
• gluteus medius
• gluteus minimus
• iliopsoas
• gastrocnemius
• soleus

BENEFITS

• Stretches hamstrings, lower back, hip extensors, and hip rotators

CAUTIONS

• Advanced degenerative joint disease

PERFECT YOUR FORM

• Slightly tuck your pelvis to help keep your spine grounded and your lower back on the floor.
• Avoid lifting your head or upper back.
• Avoid holding your breath.

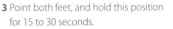

If you are feeling stiff, lie with knees bent, and then alternate lifting one leg as high and straight as you can.

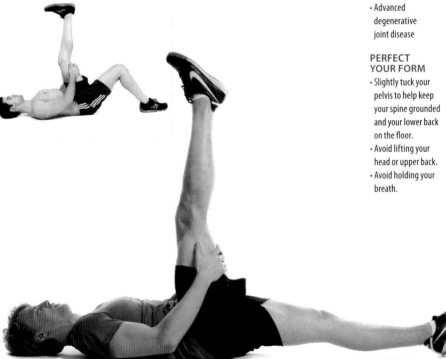

SHIN STRETCH

BEGINNER

DON'T FORGET YOUR LOWER LEG when performing a pre- or post-ride stretching session. The Shin Stretch will work the tibialis anterior at the front of your lower leg and the gastrocnemius of the back, as well as the quadriceps group at the front of your thigh.

ANNOTATION KEY

Black text indicates strengthening muscles
Gray text indicates stretching muscles
- - - - indicates deep muscles

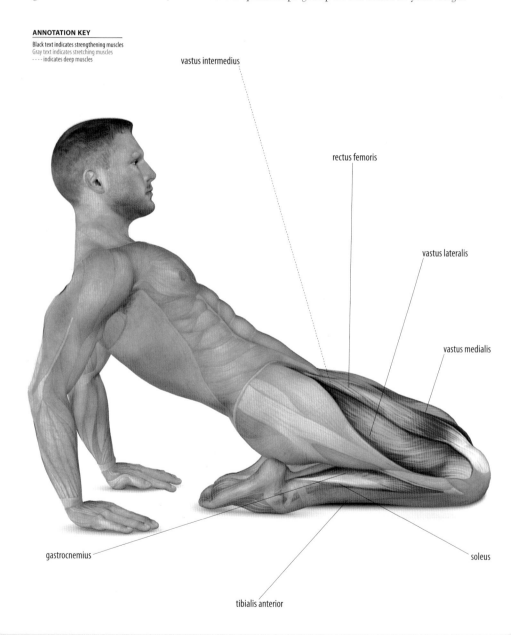

vastus intermedius

rectus femoris

vastus lateralis

vastus medialis

gastrocnemius

soleus

tibialis anterior

HOW TO DO IT

1 Kneel with your buttocks resting lightly on your heels.

2 Place your hands flat on the floor behind you with your fingers pointing forward. Keep a slight bend in your elbows.

3 Lean back slightly to increase the intensity of the stretch.

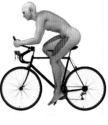

PRIMARY TARGETS

- tibialis anterior
- gastrocnemius
- soleus
- rectus femoris
- vastus lateralis
- vastus intermedius
- vastus medialis

BENEFITS

- Stretches shins and quadriceps

CAUTIONS

- Lower-back pain

PERFECT YOUR FORM

- Contract and engage your gluteal muscles to avoid a curve in your lumbar spine.
- Keep a space between your heels and glutes.
- Avoid arching your back.

HAND-TO-TOE LIFT

ADVANCED

THE HAND-TO-TOE LIFT is a versatile move that works as both a balancing and strengthening exercise for your legs and ankles while also affording the back of your legs a full stretch. Borrowed from yoga, it is a challenging stretch that you should work slowly on perfecting.

ANNOTATION KEY
Black text indicates strengthening muscles
Gray text indicates stretching muscles
- - - - indicates deep muscles

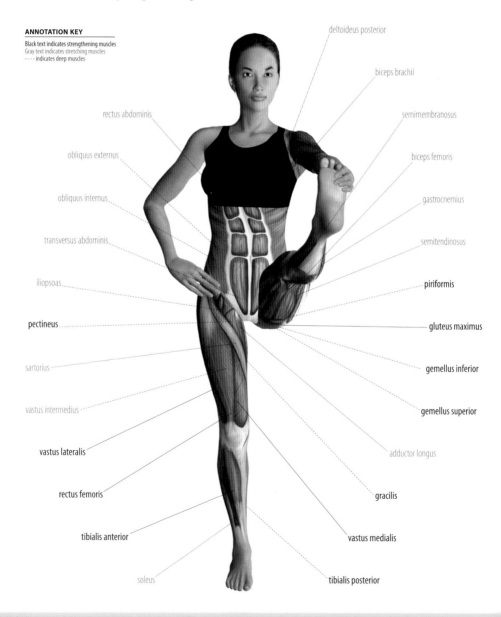

deltoideus posterior

biceps brachii

semimembranosus

rectus abdominis

obliquus externus

biceps femoris

obliquus internus

gastrocnemius

transversus abdominis

semitendinosus

iliopsoas

piriformis

pectineus

gluteus maximus

sartorius

gemellus inferior

vastus intermedius

gemellus superior

vastus lateralis

adductor longus

rectus femoris

gracilis

tibialis anterior

vastus medialis

soleus

tibialis posterior

HOW TO DO IT

1 Stand with both feet equally balanced on the floor, your shoulders relaxed but retracted back. Shift your weight onto your right foot.

2 Raise your left leg toward your chest by bending your left knee. Grasp your toes with your left hand. Rest your right hand on your right hip.

3 Extend your left leg, straightening it while pulling your foot inward as your extended leg moves to come in line with your torso.

4 Gaze at a single spot on the floor about a body's length in front of you. Flex your foot so that your toes curl back toward you. Hold for 5 seconds.

5 Lower your foot to the floor, and repeat five times on each side.

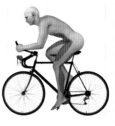

PRIMARY TARGETS
- biceps femoris
- semitendinosus
- semimembranosus
- rectus femoris
- vastus lateralis
- vastus medialis
- quadratus lumborum
- piriformis
- gemellus superior
- gemellus inferior
- tibialis anterior
- gracilis
- gluteus maximus

BENEFITS
- Improves sense of balance
- Strengthens legs and ankles
- Stretches backs of the legs

CAUTIONS
- Ankle injury
- Lower-back injury

PERFECT YOUR FORM
- Keep your hips square and facing forward—even when you raise your leg.
- Lift your torso.
- Avoid moving the hip of your raised leg toward your lower ribs so that your hips are no longer aligned.

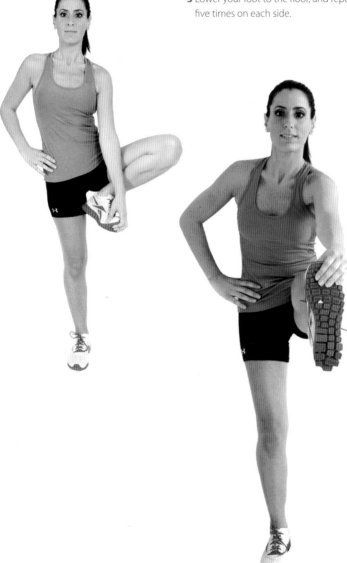

CALF STRETCH

BEGINNER

THE CALF STRETCH targets your gastrocnemius, the large bifurcated muscle at the back of your calf. It also stretches the soleus muscle and Achilles tendon.

ANNOTATION KEY
Black text indicates strengthening muscles
Gray text indicates stretching muscles
Italic text indicates tendons and ligaments
- - - - indicates deep muscles

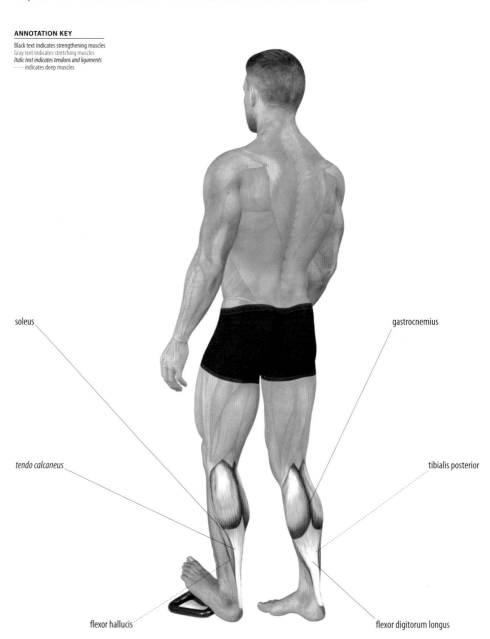

soleus

gastrocnemius

tendo calcaneus

tibialis posterior

flexor hallucis

flexor digitorum longus

HOW TO DO IT

1 Stand with your feet parallel and close together and your arms at your sides. Place a dumbbell on the floor in front of you.

2 Step forward to place the toes of your left foot on the dumbbell bar.

3 Lower your heel to the floor until you can feel a stretch.

4 Hold for 20 to 30 seconds, and repeat. Switch sides, and repeat on the right leg.

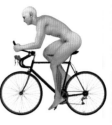

KEEPING FLEXIBLE

PRIMARY TARGETS
- gastrocnemius
- tibialis posterior
- soleus
- flexor digitorum
- flexor hallucis
- tendo calcaneus

BENEFITS
- Stretches calf muscles

CAUTIONS
- No restrictions

PERFECT YOUR FORM
- Keep your front foot anchored on the dumbbell.
- Keep your hips square.
- Avoid twisting your hips.
- Avoid arching your back or hunching forward.

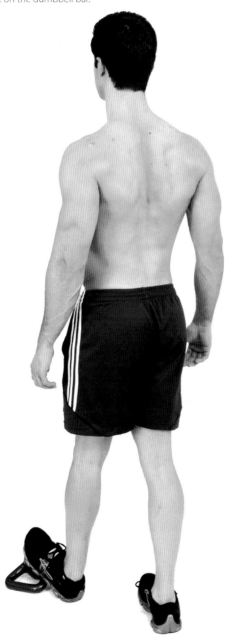

POINT & FLEX FOOT STRETCHES

BEGINNER

DON'T FORGET YOUR FEET when you are working to keep your body flexible. Stiff or tight ankles, arches, and toes can restrict your movement, making riding inefficient or even painful. A simple routine, such as performing the Point & Flex Foot Stretches regularly, can improve both the strength and flexibility of your feet, calves, and ankles.

ANNOTATION KEY

Black text indicates strengthening muscles
Gray text indicates stretching muscles
- - - - indicates deep muscles

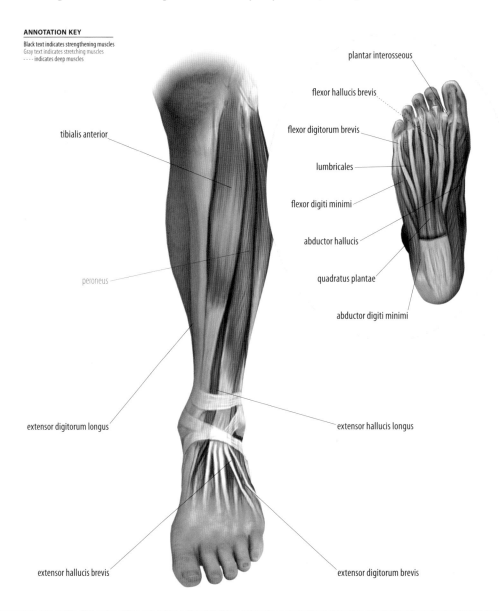

plantar interosseous

flexor hallucis brevis

flexor digitorum brevis

tibialis anterior

lumbricales

flexor digiti minimi

abductor hallucis

peroneus

quadratus plantae

abductor digiti minimi

extensor digitorum longus

extensor hallucis longus

extensor hallucis brevis

extensor digitorum brevis

HOW TO DO IT

1 Sit on a chair or mat, and cross your right leg over the left so that your ankle rests on top of your left thigh.

2 Brace your right ankle with your right hand, and grasp the front of your right foot with your left hand. Press down on the top of your foot, focusing the palm of your hand on the knuckles of your toes so that they point inward.

3 Release back to starting position.

4 While still seated with your right ankle resting on top of your left thigh, brace your right heel with your right hand, and grasp the bottom of your toes and ball of the foot with your left hand.

5 Pull back on your toes, flexing them until you feel a stretch in your arch.

6 Return to starting position, switch legs, and repeat both point and flex portions of the stretch on the other side.

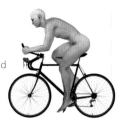

PRIMARY TARGETS

- extensor digitorum longus and brevis
- tibialis anterior
- extensor hallucis longus and brevis
- flexor digitorum longus and brevis
- quadratus plantae
- flexor digiti minimi brevis
- flexor hallucis brevis
- lumbricales
- plantar interosseous
- abductor digiti minimi
- abductor hallucis

BENEFITS

- Stretches feet, shins, and arches
- Strengthens ankles
- Improves range of motion in feet and calves
- Helps prevent soreness, cramping, and other discomfort while pedalling

CAUTIONS

- No restrictions

PERFECT YOUR FORM

- Avoid allowing your foot to shift— firmly stabilize your ankle and heel.

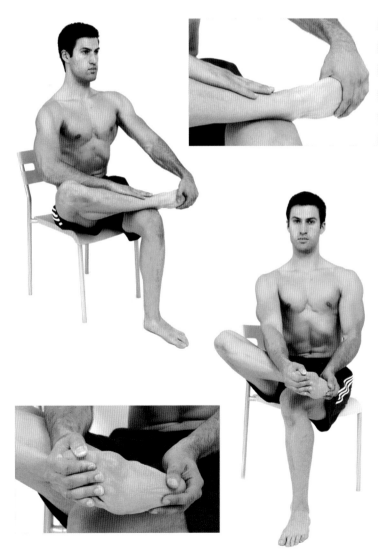

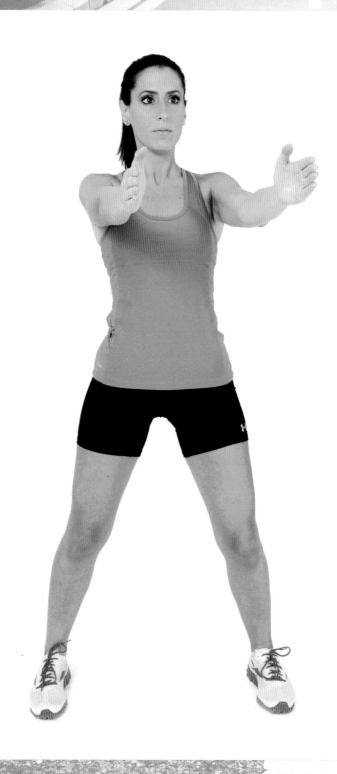

STRENGTHENING YOUR ARMS & LEGS

For cyclists, the benefits of building strong legs are evident. Strength translates naturally to power on the bike; speed is attained by pedaling faster. Without strength, important sprinting or hill-climbing skills will be lacking.

The following exercises will increase muscle strength while also contributing to the development of bone strength that a cycling-only regimen lacks. What's more, supplementing your cycling with strengthening exercises like Thigh Rock-Back or the Clamshell Series, along with weight-bearing moves like Power Squat, counteracts the dreaded "plateau" effect that can occur when you carry out the same movement exclusively and repeatedly.

The quadriceps, gluteal muscles, hamstrings, and hip flexors are the primary muscles used in cycling, while strong arm and shoulder muscles also play a role. The following exercises will help you build the strength you need to cycle to the best of your ability.

CHAIR DIP

BEGINNER

YOUR LEG MUSCLES may get most of the attention, but your arm muscles also effect how well you ride. Strong arms experience less metabolic stress as you ride, which means that you will have more energy—especially during long excursions. The Chair Dip, which targets the back of the arms, is one of the most effective triceps-toning exercises there is.

ANNOTATION KEY

Black text indicates strengthening muscles
Gray text indicates stretching muscles
indicates deep muscles

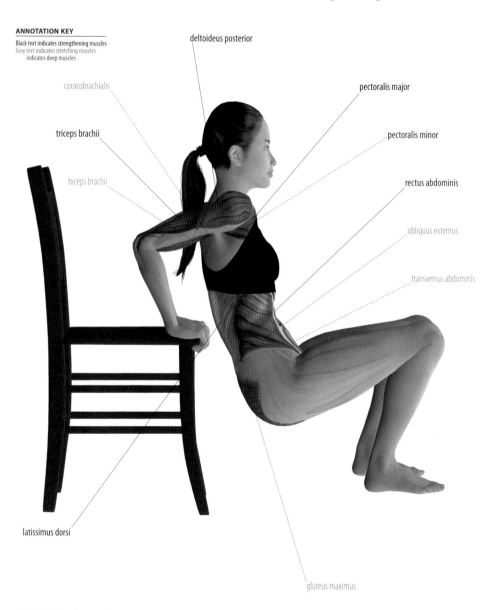

deltoideus posterior

coracobrachialis

pectoralis major

triceps brachii

pectoralis minor

biceps brachii

rectus abdominis

obliquus externus

transversus abdominis

latissimus dorsi

gluteus maximus

HOW TO DO IT

1 Sit up tall near the front of a sturdy chair. Place your hands beside your hips, wrapping your fingers over the front edge of the chair.

2 Extend your legs in front of you slightly, and place your feet flat on the floor.

3 Scoot off the edge of the chair until your knees align directly above your feet and your torso will be able to clear the chair as you dip down.

4 Bending your elbows directly behind you, without splaying them out to the sides, lower your torso until your elbows make a 90-degree angle.

5 Press into the chair, raising your body back to the starting position. Repeat 15 times for two sets.

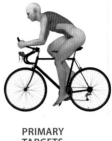

PRIMARY TARGETS
- rectus abdominis
- triceps brachii
- deltoideus posterior
- pectoralis major
- pectoralis minor
- latissimus dorsi

BENEFITS
- Strengthens your shoulder girdle
- Trains torso to remain stable while legs and arms are in motion

CAUTIONS
- Shoulder pain
- Wrist pain

PERFECT YOUR FORM
- Keep your body close to the chair.
- Keep your spine in neutral position throughout the movement.
- Avoid allowing your shoulders to lift toward your ears.
- Avoid rounding your back at your hips.
- Avoid pushing up solely with your feet rather than using your arm strength.
- Don't move your feet.

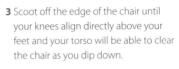
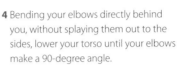
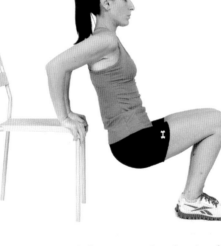
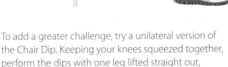

To add a greater challenge, try a unilateral version of the Chair Dip. Keeping your knees squeezed together, perform the dips with one leg lifted straight out, parallel to the floor. Repeat 15 times on each side.

PUSH-UP

BEGINNER

THE CLASSIC PUSH-UP is found in just about every workout regimen, from high school physical education to military basic training. Push-Ups target the pectoral muscles, triceps, and anterior deltoids with secondary benefits to your posterior and medial deltoids, serratus anterior, coracobrachialis, and your entire midsection.

ANNOTATION KEY

Black text indicates strengthening muscles
Gray text indicates stretching muscles
- - - - indicates deep muscles

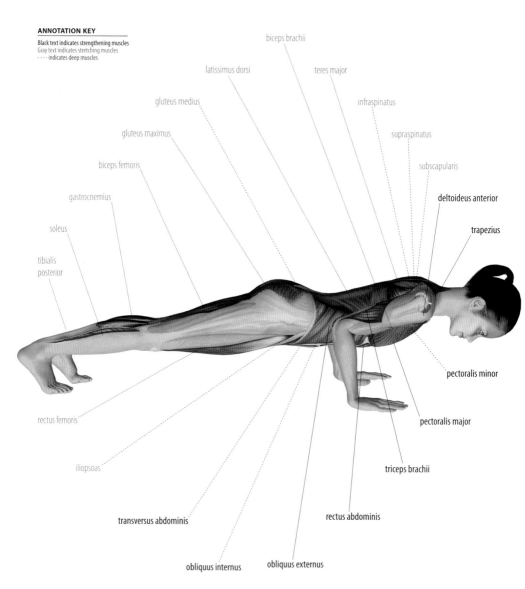

biceps brachii

latissimus dorsi

teres major

gluteus medius

infraspinatus

gluteus maximus

supraspinatus

biceps femoris

subscapularis

gastrocnemius

deltoideus anterior

soleus

trapezius

tibialis posterior

pectoralis minor

rectus femoris

pectoralis major

iliopsoas

triceps brachii

transversus abdominis

rectus abdominis

obliquus internus

obliquus externus

HOW TO DO IT

1 From a standing position, bend forward and walk your hands out until they are directly beneath your shoulders in a high plank position.

2 Inhale, and set your body by drawing your abdominals to your spine. Squeeze your buttocks and legs together and stretch out of your heels, bringing your body into a straight line.

3 Exhale and inhale as you bend your elbows and lower your body toward the floor.

4 Push upward to return to plank position. Keep your elbows close to your body. Repeat eight times.

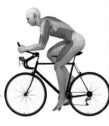

PRIMARY TARGETS

- triceps brachii
- pectoralis major
- pectoralis minor
- coracobrachialis
- deltoideus anterior
- rectus abdominis
- transversus abdominis
- obliquus externus
- obliquus internus
- trapezius

BENEFITS

- Strengthens the core stabilizers, shoulders, back, glutes, and pectoral muscles

CAUTIONS

- Shoulder issues
- Wrist pain
- Lower-back pain

PERFECT YOUR FORM

- Relax your neck, keeping it long as you perform the upward movement.
- Squeeze your glutes as you scoop in your abdominals for stability.
- Avoid allowing your shoulders to lift toward your ears.

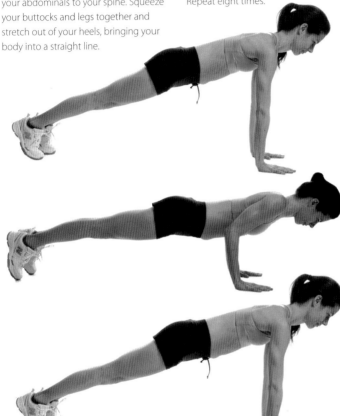

If you find a full Push-Up difficult, try this easier version: Kneel with your hands on the floor in front of you, supporting your torso. Keeping your hips open, bend and straighten your elbows as if you were going to perform a push-up.

To add a greater challenge to the Push-Up, place the balls of your feet on top of a Swiss ball while supporting your body with your hands on the floor in front of you. Use your abdominals to keep your body in a straight line and balance as you complete the push-up.

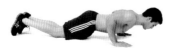

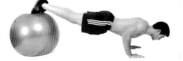

STEP-DOWN

BEGINNER

STEP-DOWN is a great strength builder for the muscles that support your knees and pelvis. Regularly performing it will improve knee control and strengthen your quads for efficient pedaling while also improving your balance and core strength.

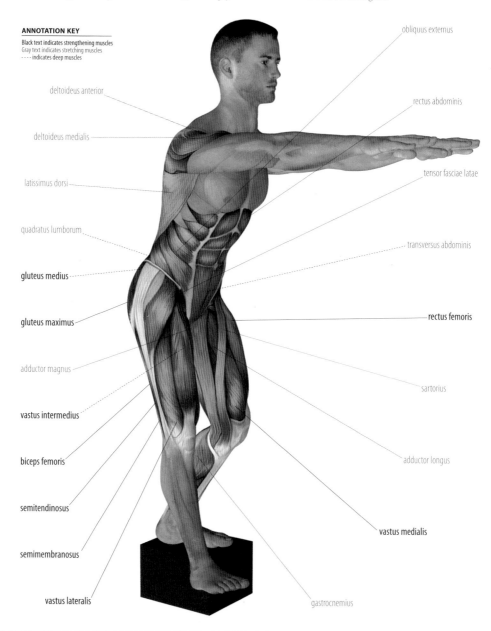

ANNOTATION KEY
Black text indicates strengthening muscles
Gray text indicates stretching muscles
---- indicates deep muscles

deltoideus anterior

deltoideus medialis

latissimus dorsi

quadratus lumborum

gluteus medius

gluteus maximus

adductor magnus

vastus intermedius

biceps femoris

semitendinosus

semimembranosus

vastus lateralis

obliquus externus

rectus abdominis

tensor fasciae latae

transversus abdominis

rectus femoris

sartorius

adductor longus

vastus medialis

gastrocnemius

HOW TO DO IT

1 Standing up straight on a firm step or block, firmly plant your left foot close to the edge, allowing your right foot to hang off the side. Flex the toes of your right foot.

2 Lift your arms out in front of you for balance, keeping them parallel to the floor. Lower your torso as you bend at your hips and knees, dropping your right leg toward the floor.

3 Without rotating your torso or knee, press upward through your left leg to return to the starting position. Repeat 15 times for two sets on each leg.

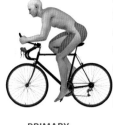

PRIMARY TARGETS
- vastus medialis
- vastus lateralis
- vastus intermedius
- rectus femoris
- gluteus maximus
- gluteus medius
- semitendinosus
- semimembranosus
- biceps femoris

BENEFITS
- Strengthens pelvic and knee stabilizers

CAUTIONS
- Ankle pain
- Sharp knee pain
- Lower-back pain

PERFECT YOUR FORM
- Align your bent knee with your second toe so that your knee doesn't rotate inward.
- Bend your knees and hips at the same time.
- Keep your hips behind your foot, leaning your torso forward as you lower into the bend.
- Avoid craning your neck.
- Avoid placing weight on the foot being lowered to the floor—only allow a light touch.

UNILATERAL LEG CIRCLES

BEGINNER

ONE OF THE BASIC EXERCISES of Pilates, Unilateral Leg Circles are an effective way to develop abdominal control while working your hip adductors, hip abductors, and quads. Working on one side at a time allows you to focus on multiple muscle groups.

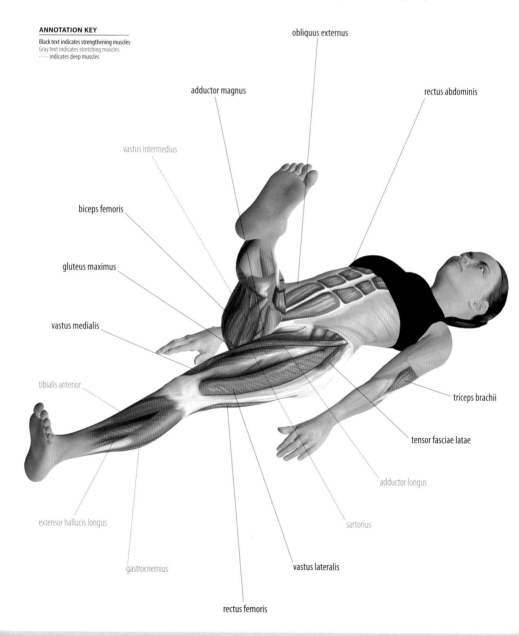

ANNOTATION KEY

Black text indicates strengthening muscles
Gray text indicates stretching muscles
- - - - indicates deep muscles

obliquus externus

adductor magnus

rectus abdominis

vastus intermedius

biceps femoris

gluteus maximus

vastus medialis

tibialis anterior

triceps brachii

tensor fasciae latae

adductor longus

extensor hallucis longus

sartorius

gastrocnemius

vastus lateralis

rectus femoris

HOW TO DO IT

1 Lie flat on the floor with both arms and legs extended

2 Bend your right knee toward your chest, and then straighten your right leg up in the air. Anchor the rest of your body to the floor, straightening both knees and pressing your shoulders back and down.

3 Cross your raised leg up and over your body, aiming for your left shoulder.

4 Continue making a circle with the raised leg, returning to the center. Add emphasis to the motion by pausing at the top between repetitions.

5 Switch directions, and repeat. Lower your leg, and then repeat with the other leg. Complete full movement five to eight times.

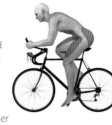

PRIMARY TARGETS
- rectus abdominis
- obliquus externus
- rectus femoris
- biceps femoris
- triceps brachii
- gluteus maximus
- adductor magnus
- vastus lateralis
- vastus medialis
- tensor fasciae latae

BENEFITS
- Lengthens leg muscles
- Stabilizes pelvis
- Strengthens deep abdominal muscles

CAUTIONS
- Snapping hip syndrome—if this is an issue, reduce the size of the circles.

PERFECT YOUR FORM
- Keep your hips and torso stable while your legs are mobilized.
- Elongate your raised leg from your hip through your foot.
- Avoid making your leg circles too big to maintain stability.

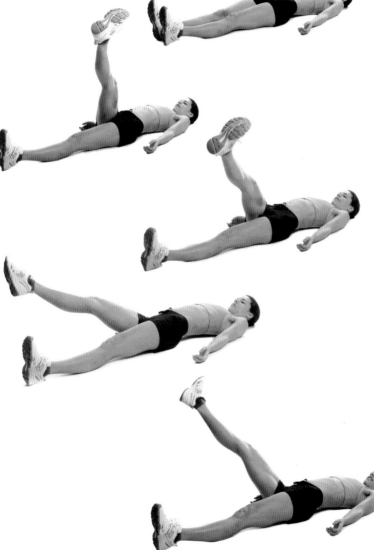

LATERAL LOW LUNGE

BEGINNER

THE LATERAL LOW LUNGE, also known as a Side Lunge, increases the mobility of your hips and loosens the muscles of your glutes and groins while opening up your calves, quads, hamstrings, lateral thighs, and hips.

ANNOTATION KEY
Black text indicates strengthening muscles
Gray text indicates stretching muscles
- - - - indicates deep muscles

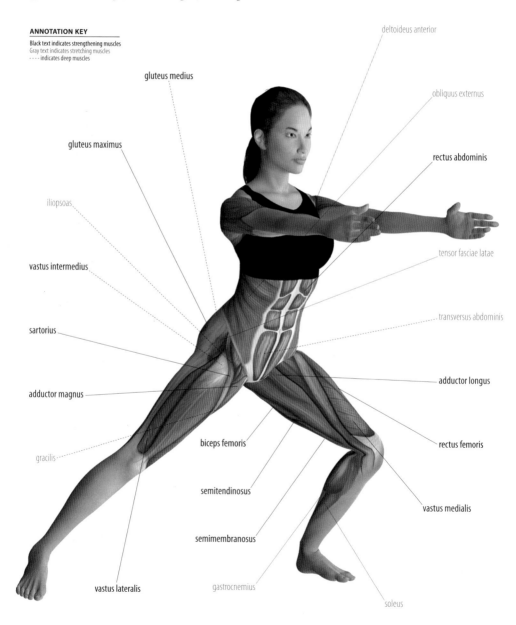

deltoideus anterior

gluteus medius

obliquus externus

gluteus maximus

rectus abdominis

iliopsoas

vastus intermedius

tensor fasciae latae

transversus abdominis

sartorius

adductor longus

adductor magnus

biceps femoris

rectus femoris

gracilis

semitendinosus

vastus medialis

semimembranosus

vastus lateralis

gastrocnemius

soleus

HOW TO DO IT

1 Stand with your feet planted widely and your arms outstretched in front of you, parallel to the floor.

2 Step out to the left. Squat down on your left leg, bending at your hips while maintaining a neutral spine. Begin to extend your right leg, keeping both feet flat on the floor.

3 Bend your left knee until your thigh is parallel to the floor, and your right leg is fully extended.

4 Keeping your arms parallel to the floor, squeeze your buttocks and press off your left leg to return to the starting position, and repeat. Repeat sequence 10 times on each side.

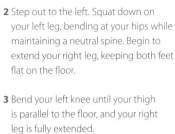
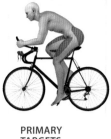

PRIMARY TARGETS

- adductor longus
- adductor magnus
- semitendinosus
- semimembranosus
- biceps femoris
- sartorius
- vastus medialis
- vastus lateralis
- vastus intermedius
- rectus femoris
- gluteus maximus
- gluteus medius
- rectus abdominis

BENEFITS

- Strengthens the trunk, knee, and pelvic stabilizers

CAUTIONS

- Knee pain
- Back pain
- Trouble bearing weight on one leg

PERFECT YOUR FORM

- Keep your spine in neutral position as you bend your hips.
- Relax your neck and shoulders.
- Align your knee with the toe of your bent leg.
- Tighten your glutes as you bend.
- Avoid craning your neck as you perform the movement.
- Avoid lifting your feet off the floor.
- Avoid arching or extending your back.

STRENGTHENING YOUR ARMS & LEGS

YOGA LUNGE

BEGINNER

THIS VERSION OF A FORWARD LUNGE is usually called High Lunge in yoga, but it is also known as a low forward lunge. It is an effective leg and arm strengthener that targets your glutes and quadriceps, along with your hamstrings, soleus, and gastrocnemius muscles. The deep position will also stretch your groins.

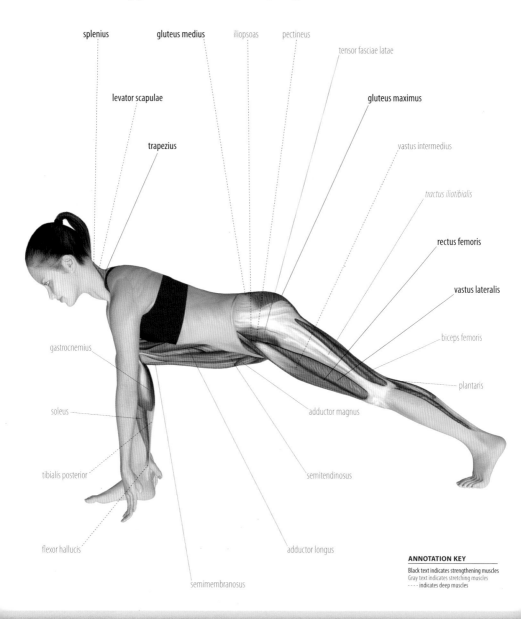

splenius

gluteus medius

iliopsoas

pectineus

tensor fasciae latae

levator scapulae

gluteus maximus

trapezius

vastus intermedius

tractus iliotibialis

rectus femoris

vastus lateralis

gastrocnemius

biceps femoris

plantaris

soleus

adductor magnus

tibialis posterior

semitendinosus

flexor hallucis

adductor longus

semimembranosus

ANNOTATION KEY
Black text indicates strengthening muscles
Gray text indicates stretching muscles
- - - - indicates deep muscles

HOW TO DO IT

1 Stand with your feet together and your arms hanging at your sides.

2 Exhale, and carefully step back with your left leg, keeping it in line with your hips as you step back. The ball of your right foot should be in contact with the floor as you do the motion.

3 Slowly slide your left foot farther back while bending your right knee, stacking it directly above your ankle.

4 Position your palms or fingertips on the floor on either side of your right leg, and slowly press your palms or fingertips against the floor to enhance the placement of your upper body and your head.

5 Lift your head and gaze straight forward while leaning your upper body forward and carefully rolling your shoulders downward and back.

6 Press the ball of your right foot gradually into the floor, contract your thigh muscles, and press up to keep your left leg straight.

7 Hold for 5 seconds. Slowly return to the starting position, and then repeat on the other side.

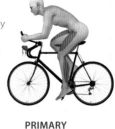

PRIMARY TARGETS

- biceps femoris
- adductor longus
- adductor magnus
- gastrocnemius
- tibialis posterior
- iliopsoas
- biceps femoris
- rectus femoris

BENEFITS

- Strengthens legs and arms
- Stretches groins

CAUTIONS

- Arm injury
- Shoulder injury
- Hip injury
- High or low blood pressure
- Severe headache

PERFECT YOUR FORM

- Maintain proper position of your shoulders and your whole upper body to lengthen your spine.
- Avoid dropping your back-extended knee to the floor.

HEEL BEATS

BEGINNER

HEEL BEATS, one of the classical Pilates mat exercises, is a multipurpose exercise that tones and strengthens your muscles from the back of your neck to the tendons of your feet, including your abdominals, inner thighs, and hamstrings. It is also a phenomenal exercise for firming your glutes, giving them an enviable raised and rounded look.

ANNOTATION KEY

Black text indicates strengthening muscles
Gray text indicates stretching muscles
- - - - indicates deep muscles

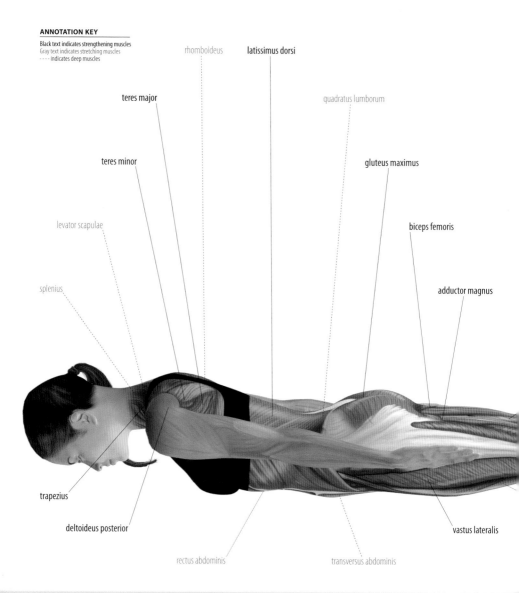

rhomboideus

latissimus dorsi

teres major

quadratus lumborum

teres minor

gluteus maximus

levator scapulae

biceps femoris

splenius

adductor magnus

trapezius

deltoideus posterior

rectus abdominis

transversus abdominis

vastus lateralis

HOW TO DO IT

1 Lie facedown with your arms lifted off the floor by your hips, palms up. Draw your shoulders down away from your ears. Turn your legs out from the top of your hips and pull your inner thighs together.

2 Pull your navel off the mat and toward your spine, pressing your pubic bone into the mat. Lengthen your legs and lift them off the mat, tightening your thigh muscles.

3 Press your heels together, allowing them to lightly touch, and then separate them in a rapid but controlled motion.

4 Beat heels together for eight counts, then return to the starting position. Repeat sequence six to eight times.

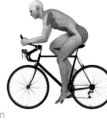

PRIMARY TARGETS
- teres major
- teres minor
- deltoideus posterior
- trapezius
- latissimus dorsi
- gluteus maximus
- biceps femoris
- adductor magnus
- soleus
- vastus lateralis

BENEFITS
- Encourages muscles from the entire body to work together
- Lengthens extensors

CAUTIONS
- Back pain

PERFECT YOUR FORM
- Squeeze your buttocks and your abdominals while beating your heels.
- Keep your breathing calm and steady.
- Avoid tensing your shoulders.

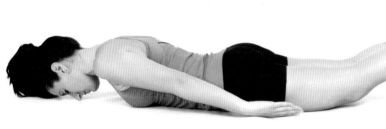

semitendinosus

gastrocnemius

peroneus

soleus

tibialis anterior

semimembranosus

rectus femoris

WALL SIT

INTERMEDIATE

THE WALL SIT is an excellent isometric exercise that targets the all-important quads, glutes, and calves. In an isometric exercise, the contracting muscles produce little or no movement, but you'll gain leg strength and endurance for long-distance riding.

ANNOTATION KEY

Black text indicates strengthening muscles
Gray text indicates stretching muscles
- - - - indicates deep muscles

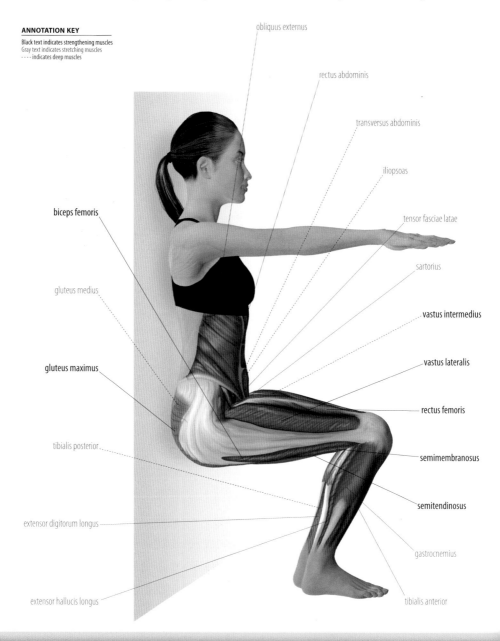

obliquus externus

rectus abdominis

transversus abdominis

iliopsoas

tensor fasciae latae

sartorius

biceps femoris

gluteus medius

vastus intermedius

vastus lateralis

gluteus maximus

rectus femoris

tibialis posterior

semimembranosus

semitendinosus

extensor digitorum longus

gastrocnemius

extensor hallucis longus

tibialis anterior

HOW TO DO IT

1 Stand with your back to a wall. Lean against the wall, and walk your feet out from under your body until your lower back rests comfortably against it.

2 Slide your torso down the wall, until your hips and knees form 90-degree angles, your thighs parallel to the floor.

3 Raise your arms straight in front of you so that they are parallel to your thighs, and relax your upper torso. Hold for 1 minute, and then return to the starting position. Repeat five times.

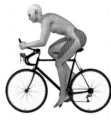

PRIMARY TARGETS
- vastus medialis
- vastus lateralis
- vastus intermedius
- rectus femoris
- semitendinosus
- semimembranosus
- biceps femoris
- gluteus maximus

BENEFITS
- Strengthens glutes and quadriceps
- Trains the body to place weight evenly between the legs

CAUTIONS
- Knee pain

PERFECT YOUR FORM
- Keep your body firm throughout the exercise.
- Relax your neck and shoulders.
- Form a 90-degree angle with your hips and knees to receive maximum benefit from the exercise.
- Avoid sitting below 90 degrees.
- Don't push your back into the wall to hold yourself up.
- Avoid shifting from side to side as you begin to fatigue.

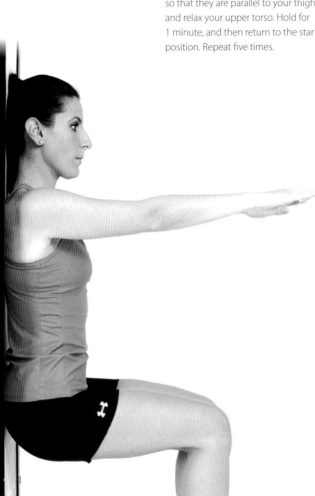

STRENGTHENING YOUR ARMS & LEGS

CLAMSHELL SERIES

INTERMEDIATE

THE CLAMSHELL SERIES utilizes hip external rotation to effectively work your glutes while also working much of your legs, especially the hamstrings at the backs of your thighs. Use this exercise to develop a stronger back and stable knees, which promote better cycling form.

ANNOTATION KEY

Black text indicates strengthening muscles
Gray text indicates stretching muscles
---- indicates deep muscles

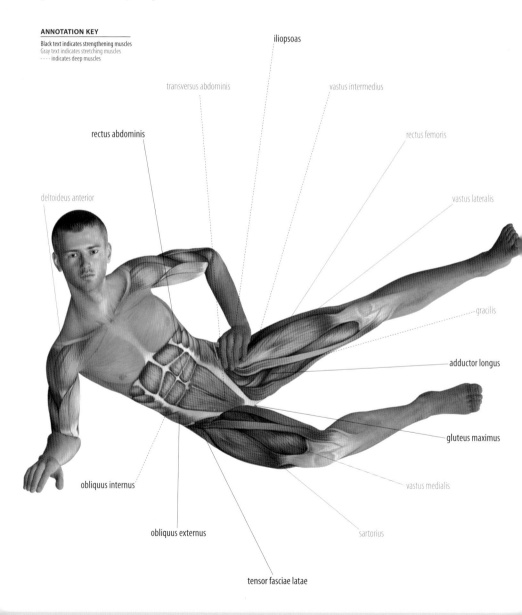

iliopsoas

transversus abdominis

vastus intermedius

rectus abdominis

rectus femoris

deltoideus anterior

vastus lateralis

gracilis

adductor longus

gluteus maximus

obliquus internus

vastus medialis

obliquus externus

sartorius

tensor fasciae latae

HOW TO DO IT

1 Lie on your right side with knees bent and legs stacked on top of each other. Bend your left elbow, placing it directly underneath your shoulder so that your forearm is supporting your upper body. Place your left hand on your hip.

2 Without moving your hips, open your left knee upward, and then return to the starting position. Repeat 10 times.

3 Lift both ankles off the floor, making sure to maintain a straight line with your torso.

4 While your ankles are still lifted, lift and lower your left knee to open and close your legs. Repeat 10 times.

5 The final part of this series begins with both ankles elevated. Lift your left knee to separate your legs, and then straighten your left leg, being careful not to move the position of your thigh. Bend your knee and return to the starting position. Repeat 10 times, switch sides, and start from the beginning.

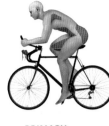

PRIMARY TARGETS
- rectus abdominis
- obliquus internus
- obliquus externus
- tensor fasciae latae
- adductor magnus
- adductor longus
- iliopsoas
- gluteus medius
- gluteus minimus
- gluteus maximus
- quadratus lumborum

BENEFITS
- Strengthens glutes
- Stabilizes pelvis
- Strengthens hip abductor muscles
- Targets shoulder stabilizers for strengthening and endurance

CAUTIONS
- Shoulder injury
- Lower-back pain or injury

PERFECT YOUR FORM
- Stack your hips and pull them forward slightly.
- Press your shoulder and forearm into the floor throughout the exercise.
- Relax your neck and shoulders.
- Avoid allowing your hips to move while lifting your knee.

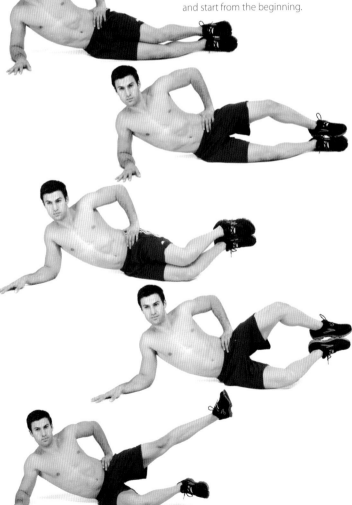

PLANK ROLL-DOWN

INTERMEDIATE

THE PLANK ROLL-DOWN is a Pilates exercise that combines the benefits of the Plank and the Push-Up to strengthen your arms, chest, and abdominals. Control is more important than the number of repetitions you can perform, so concentrate on the quality of your movements rather than the quantity.

ANNOTATION KEY

Black text indicates strengthening muscles
Gray text indicates stretching muscles
- - - - indicates deep muscles

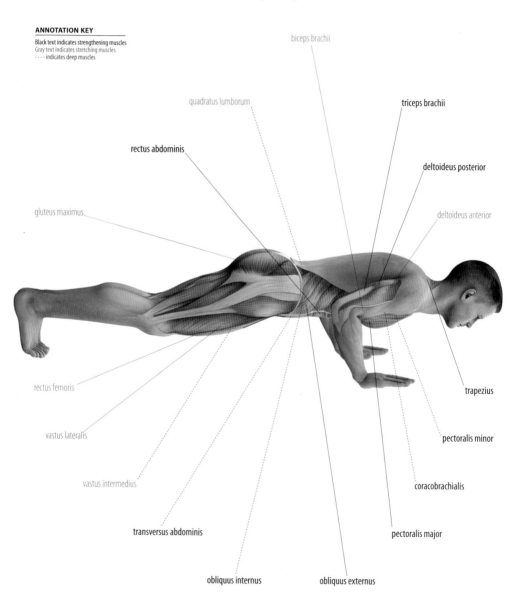

biceps brachii

quadratus lumborum

triceps brachii

rectus abdominis

deltoideus posterior

deltoideus anterior

gluteus maximus

rectus femoris

trapezius

vastus lateralis

pectoralis minor

vastus intermedius

coracobrachialis

transversus abdominis

pectoralis major

obliquus internus

obliquus externus

HOW TO DO IT

1 Stand straight, inhale, and pull your navel to your spine.

2 Exhale as you roll down one vertebra at a time until your hands touch the floor in front of you.

3 Walk your hands out until they are directly beneath your shoulders in the plank position.

4 Inhale, and "set" your body by drawing your abdominals toward your spine. Squeeze your buttocks and legs together and stretch out of your heels, bringing your body into a straight line.

5 Exhale and inhale as you bend your elbows and lower your body toward the floor. Then push upward to return to plank position. Keep your elbows close to your body. Repeat eight times.

6 Inhale as you lift your hips upward, and walk your hands back toward your feet. Exhale slowly, rolling up one vertebra at a time into your starting position. Repeat the entire exercise three times.

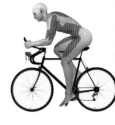

PRIMARY TARGETS
- triceps brachii
- pectoralis major
- pectoralis minor
- coracobrachialis
- deltoideus posterior
- rectus abdominis
- transversus abdominis
- obliquus externus
- obliquus internus
- trapezius

BENEFITS
- Strengthens shoulders, pectoral muscles, core stabilizers, back, and glutes

CAUTIONS
- Shoulder issues
- Wrist pain
- Lower-back pain

PERFECT YOUR FORM
- Keep your neck long and relaxed.
- Tightly squeeze your glutes you scoop in your abdominals for stability.
- Avoid allowing your shoulders to lift toward your ears.

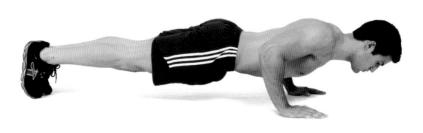
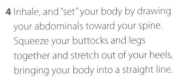
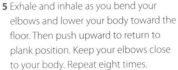

PLANK PRESS-UP

INTERMEDIATE

TO PREPARE YOUR ARMS for the endurance test of a long ride, perform the Plank Press-Up, which gives your arms and shoulders an intense workout. Focus on balance and control to avoid overextending your shoulders. Keep an even, steady pace, with your shoulders open, making sure not to let your middle collapse.

ANNOTATION KEY

Black text indicates strengthening muscles
Gray text indicates stretching muscles
- - - - indicates deep muscles

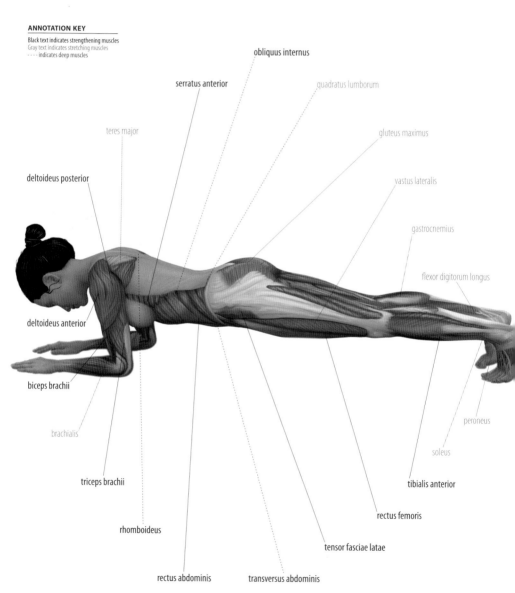

obliquus internus

serratus anterior

quadratus lumborum

teres major

gluteus maximus

deltoideus posterior

vastus lateralis

gastrocnemius

flexor digitorum longus

deltoideus anterior

biceps brachii

peroneus

brachialis

soleus

triceps brachii

tibialis anterior

rectus femoris

rhomboideus

tensor fasciae latae

rectus abdominis

transversus abdominis

HOW TO DO IT

1 Lie prone on the mat, and with your forearms underneath your chest, press your body up into a plank position, lengthening through your heels.

2 Push through your forearms to bring your shoulders up toward the ceiling.

3 Slowly, and with control, lower your shoulders until you feel them coming together in your back.

4 Repeat five times.

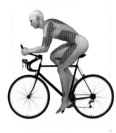

PRIMARY TARGETS

- deltoideus anterior
- deltoideus posterior
- rhomboideus
- biceps brachii
- triceps brachii
- tensor fasciae latae
- rectus femoris
- rectus abdominis
- transversus abdominis
- obliquus internus
- serratus anterior
- tibialis anterior

BENEFITS

- Strengthens scapular stabilizers
- Strengthens and stabilizes core
- Strengthens triceps
- Improves posture

CAUTIONS

- Shoulder injury
- Intense back pain

PERFECT YOUR FORM

- Avoid allowing your back to sag.
- Avoid allowing your shoulders to collapse into your shoulder joints.

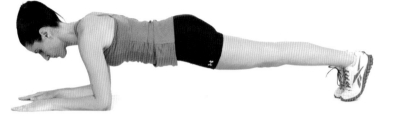

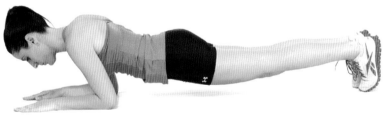

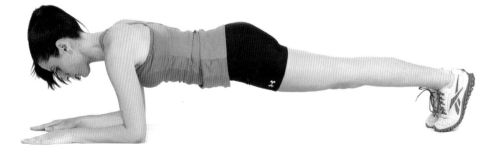

FOAM ROLLER PUSH-UP

ADVANCED

THE FOAM ROLLER PUSH-UP adds an extra challenge to this exercise classic. Like a regular Push-Up, it targets your chest, arms, and shoulders while the addition of the foam roller provides an element of instability, which really challenges your sense of balance and coordination.

ANNOTATION KEY
Black text indicates strengthening muscles
Gray text indicates stretching muscles
---- indicates deep muscles

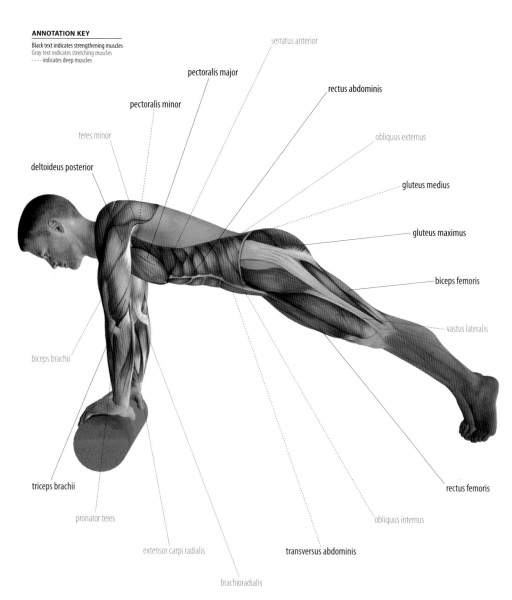

serratus anterior

pectoralis major

rectus abdominis

pectoralis minor

teres minor

obliquus externus

deltoideus posterior

gluteus medius

gluteus maximus

biceps femoris

vastus lateralis

biceps brachii

triceps brachii

rectus femoris

pronator teres

extensor carpi radialis

obliquus internus

transversus abdominis

brachioradialis

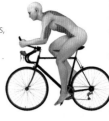

HOW TO DO IT

1 Kneel on the floor with the roller placed crosswise in front of you. Place your hands on the roller with your fingers pointed away from you.

2 Press into a plank position, lifting your knees and straightening your legs.

3 Keep your hips level with your shoulders, and without allowing your shoulders to sink, bend your elbows and lower your chest to the roller. Avoid any roller movement throughout the motion.

4 Return to the starting position by pressing upward, straightening your elbows, and maintaining a straight spine. Repeat 15 times for two sets.

PRIMARY TARGETS
- rectus abdominis
- transversus abdominis
- triceps brachii
- deltoideus posterior
- pectoralis major
- pectoralis minor
- gluteus maximus
- gluteus medius
- rectus femoris
- biceps femoris

BENEFITS
- Improves core, pelvic, and shoulder stability

CAUTIONS
- Wrist pain
- Shoulder pain
- Lower-back pain

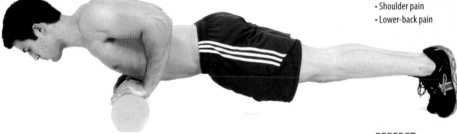

You can also perform the Push-Up on a Swiss ball. Place your hands on the ball, shoulder-width apart. With the balls of your feet on the floor behind you, complete the push-up movement while maintaining stability on the ball.

PERFECT YOUR FORM
- Look for a single plane of movement with your body forming a straight line from your shoulders to ankles.
- Relax your neck and shoulders.
- Avoid allowing your shoulders to lift toward your ears.
- Avoid raising or lowering your body in segments.
- Avoid bending your knees.

FOAM ROLLER TRICEPS DIP

ADVANCED

THE FOAM ROLLER TRICEPS DIP adds a new spin to the basic gym exercise, providing an intense workout for the hard-to-reach triceps. Balancing on the foam roller will also help you develop greater core, pelvic, and shoulder stability.

ANNOTATION KEY

Black text indicates strengthening muscles
Gray text indicates stretching muscles
- - - - indicates deep muscles

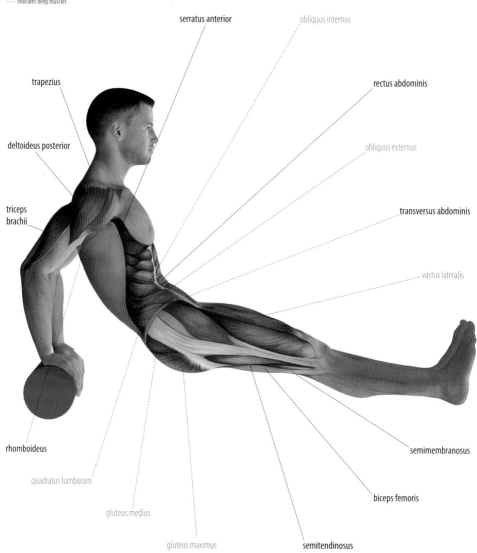

serratus anterior

obliquus internus

trapezius

rectus abdominis

deltoideus posterior

obliquus externus

triceps brachii

transversus abdominis

vastus lateralis

rhomboideus

semimembranosus

quadratus lumborum

biceps femoris

gluteus medius

gluteus maximus

semitendinosus

HOW TO DO IT

1 Sit on the floor with your legs outstretched, the foam roller behind you. Place both hands on the foam roller with your fingers facing toward your buttocks, elbows bent.

2 Press through your legs and straighten your arms to lift your hips and shoulders.

3 Keeping your shoulders pressed down away from your ears, bend your elbows and dip your trunk up and down. The foam roller should not move. Repeat 15 times for two sets.

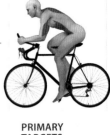

PRIMARY TARGETS

- triceps brachii
- trapezius
- rhomboideus
- deltoideus posterior
- rectus abdominis
- transversus abdominis
- serratus anterior
- biceps femoris
- semitendinosus
- semimembranosus

BENEFITS

- Improves core, pelvic, and shoulder stability

CAUTIONS

- Wrist pain
- Shoulder pain
- Discomfort in the back of the knee or knee swelling

PERFECT YOUR FORM

- Keep your legs firm with your knees straight.
- Relax your neck and shoulders.
- Firmly press the roller to the floor.
- Avoid allowing your shoulders to lift toward your ears.
- Avoid shifting the roller as you move up and down.

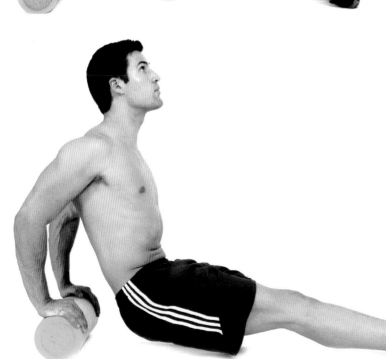

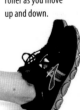

STRENGTHENING YOUR ARMS & LEGS

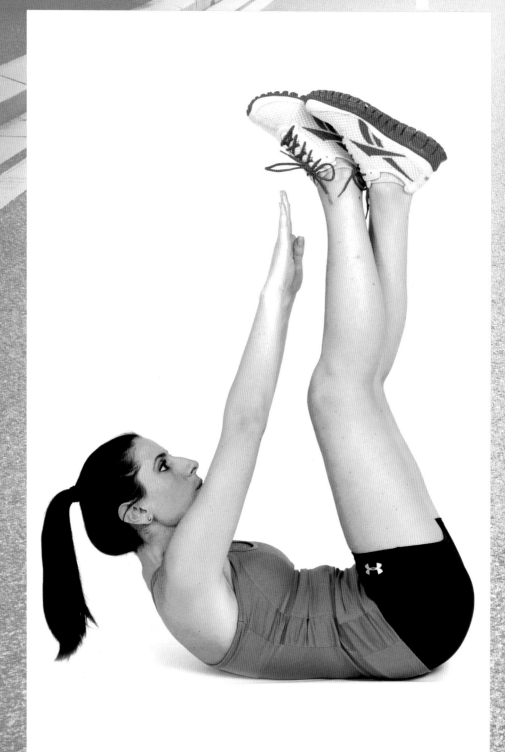

BUILDING CORE STRENGTH & STABILITY

Although cycling may seem to be all about your legs, having a strong and stable core is essential, too. When you cycle, the muscles around your pelvis, abdomen, hips, and lower back work together to contribute to a fluid pedal stroke. When these muscles are all balanced and working in concert, energy is isolated and focused through the body to the pedal, allowing you to ride with efficiency.

Your body is designed to stabilize before it engages in action, and these exercises will develop your body's ability to stabilize around your spine, which will ultimately bring about overall stability. When your core muscles are strong and engaged, your body naturally aligns to an effective and more powerful pedaling action.

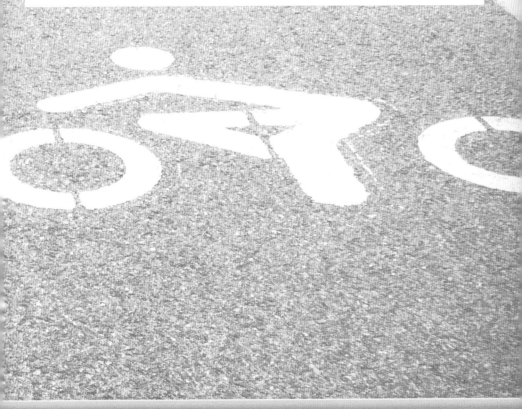

THIGH ROCK-BACK

BEGINNER

A QUADRICEPS AND ABDOMINAL STRENGTHENER, the Thigh Rock-Back also stretches your legs and ankles. Focus on controlled movement, gradually building up your strength and endurance so that you will be able to lean farther back as you reach a higher skill level.

ANNOTATION KEY

Black text indicates strengthening muscles
Gray text indicates stretching muscles
- - - - indicates deep muscles

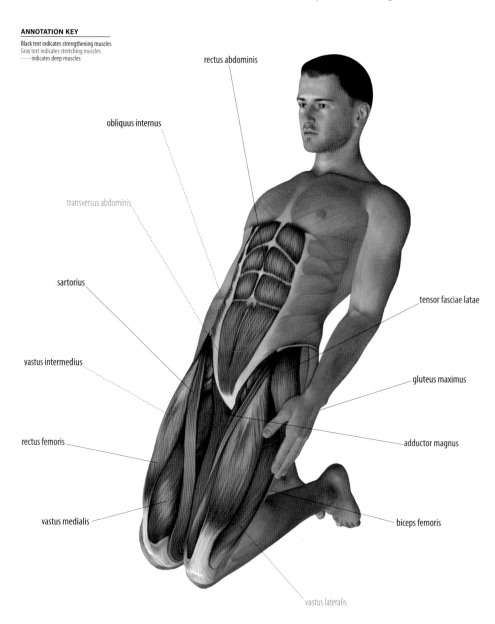

rectus abdominis

obliquus internus

transversus abdominis

sartorius

vastus intermedius

rectus femoris

vastus medialis

tensor fasciae latae

gluteus maximus

adductor magnus

biceps femoris

vastus lateralis

HOW TO DO IT

1 Kneel with your back straight and your knees hip-width apart on the floor, your arms by your sides. Pull in your abdominals, drawing your navel toward your spine.

2 Lean back, keeping your hips open and aligned with your shoulders, stretching the front of your thighs.

3 Once you have leaned back as far as you can, squeeze your buttocks and slowly bring your body back to the upright position. Repeat four to five times.

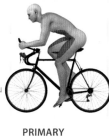

PRIMARY TARGETS

- rectus abdominis
- rectus femoris
- vastus intermedius
- vastus medialis
- tensor fasciae latae
- gluteus maximus
- adductor magnus
- sartorius
- biceps femoris
- obliquus internus

BENEFITS

- Strengthens abdominals
- Increases range of motion of anterior ankle
- Stretches thighs

CAUTIONS

- Quadriceps pain or injury

PERFECT YOUR FORM

- Form a straight line between your torso and your knees.
- Use your abdominals to control the movement.
- Tightly squeeze your glutes.
- Avoid rocking your torso back so far that you can't return to the starting position.
- Avoid bending in your hips.

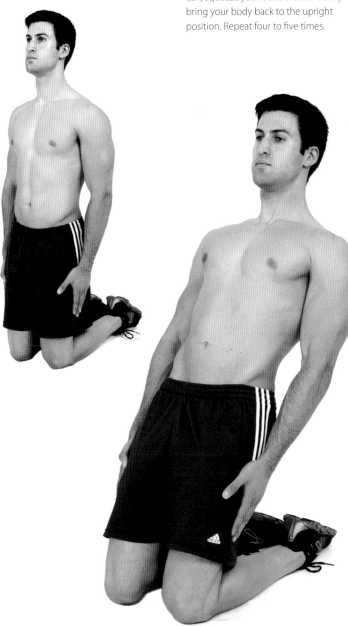

SCISSORS

INTERMEDIATE

THE SCISSORS IS ONE of the most popular of the Pilates exercises, a discipline known for its core-strengthening effects. While also working your leg muscles, this exercise helps you develop better bodily coordination.

ANNOTATION KEY

Black text indicates strengthening muscles
Gray text indicates stretching muscles
---- indicates deep muscles

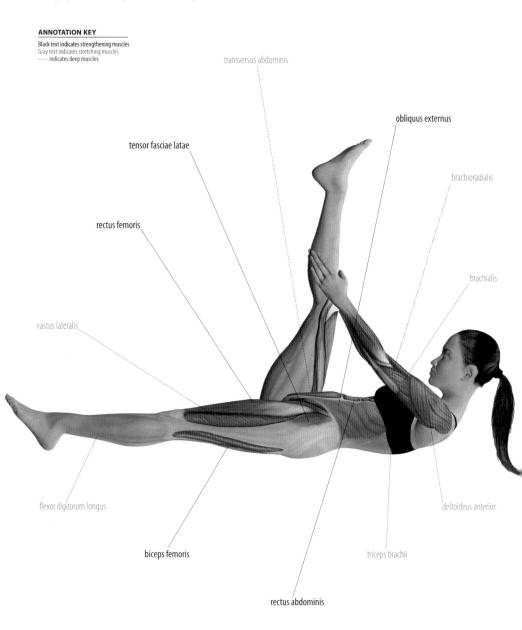

transversus abdominis

obliquus externus

tensor fasciae latae

brachioradialis

rectus femoris

brachialis

vastus lateralis

flexor digitorum longus

deltoideus anterior

biceps femoris

triceps brachii

rectus abdominis

HOW TO DO IT

1 Lie with your back on the floor, your arms by your sides, and your legs raised in a tabletop position. Inhale, drawing in your abdominals.

2 Lower your right leg as you raise your left leg toward your trunk. Hold your left calf with your hands, pulsing twice while keeping your shoulders down.

3 Switch your legs in the air, reaching for your right leg. Stabilize your pelvis and spine. Repeat sequence six to eight times on each leg.

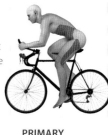

PRIMARY TARGETS
- rectus abdominis
- obliquus externus
- biceps femoris
- rectus femoris
- tensor fasciae latae

BENEFITS
- Increases abdominal strength and endurance
- Increases stability with unilateral movement

CAUTIONS
- Hamstring injury

PERFECT YOUR FORM
- Keep your legs as straight as possible.
- Draw your navel into your spine.
- If your hamstrings are tight, you may bend the knee that is moving toward your chest.
- Avoid bending your leg.

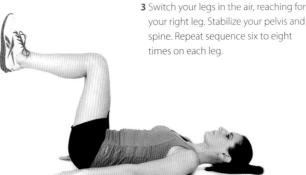

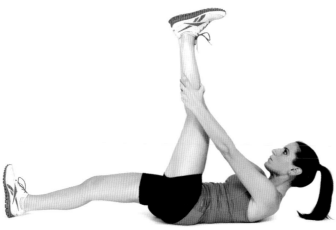

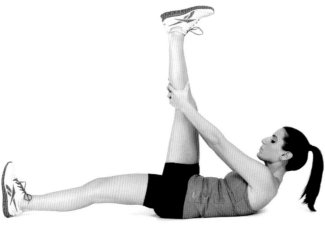

CROSSOVER CRUNCH

INTERMEDIATE

THE CROSSOVER CRUNCH targets the oblique muscles, which not only helps define your waist but strengthens and stabilizes your core so that you can cycle with the best form possible. Adding this exercise to your regimen will leave you with abdominals that are more toned and a back that has greater rotational flexibility.

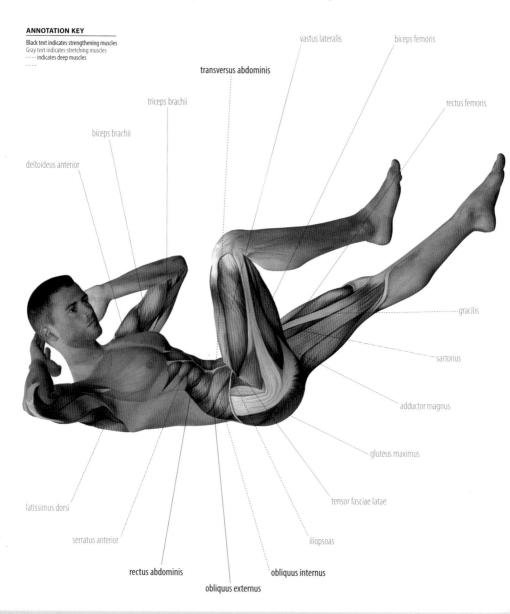

ANNOTATION KEY
Black text indicates strengthening muscles
Gray text indicates stretching muscles
----indicates deep muscles
- - - -

vastus lateralis

biceps femoris

transversus abdominis

rectus femoris

triceps brachii

biceps brachii

deltoideus anterior

gracilis

sartorius

adductor magnus

gluteus maximus

tensor fasciae latae

latissimus dorsi

iliopsoas

serratus anterior

rectus abdominis

obliquus internus

obliquus externus

HOW TO DO IT

1 Lie on your back with your hands behind your head. Lift your legs into a tabletop position, so that your thighs and calves form a 90-degree angle with your calves parallel to the floor.

For an easier variation, begin with both feet on the floor. Place the outside of one foot on top of your thigh near your knee. Reach your opposite elbow toward the knee of your raised leg.

2 Roll up with your torso, reaching your right elbow to your left knee and extending your right leg in front of you. Imagine pulling your shoulder blades off the floor and twisting from your ribs and oblique muscles.

3 Alternate extending your right and left legs. Repeat sequence six times.

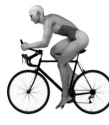

PRIMARY TARGETS
• rectus abdominis
• transversus abdominis
• obliquus externus
• obliquus internus

BENEFITS
• Stabilizes core
• Strengthens abdominals

CAUTIONS
• Neck issues
• Lower-back pain

PERFECT YOUR FORM
• Elongate your neck.
• Lift your chin away from your chest.
• Keep both hips stable on the floor.
• Avoid pulling with your hands.
• Avoid arching your back.
• Avoid moving the active elbow faster than your shoulder.

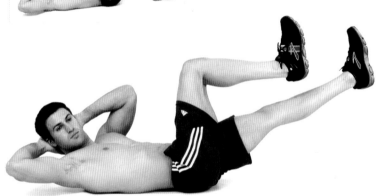

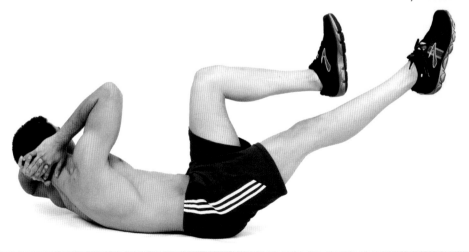

LEMON SQUEEZER

INTERMEDIATE

THE LEMON SQUEEZER is a high-intensity move that targets your abdominals and your thigh muscles. Named for the kitchen device that squeezes the juice from citrus fruit, the exercise calls for you to isolate and strongly contract your upper abdominals—as if you were squeezing a gigantic lemon between your thighs and abdominals.

ANNOTATION KEY
Black text indicates strengthening muscles
Gray text indicates stretching muscles
- - - - indicates deep muscles

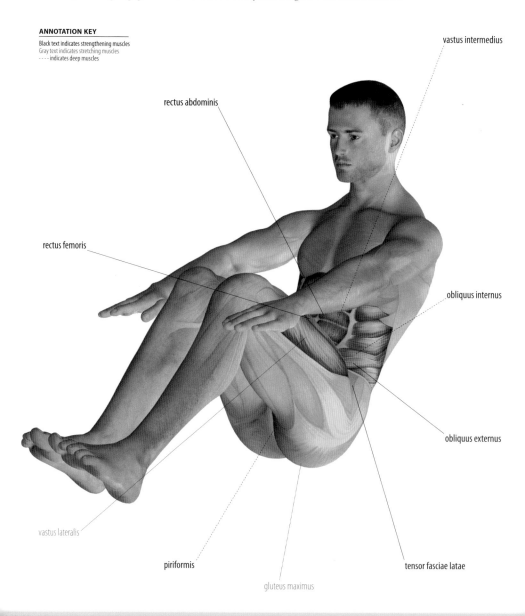

vastus intermedius

rectus abdominis

rectus femoris

obliquus internus

obliquus externus

vastus lateralis

piriformis

gluteus maximus

tensor fasciae latae

HOW TO DO IT

1 Lie supine on the floor. Lift your legs, head, neck, and shoulders slightly off the floor, being careful not to arch your lower back. Your arms should be raised and parallel to the floor.

2 Pulling your knees in toward your chest, reach your arms forward to your ankles, so that your torso lifts completely off the floor.

3 Slowly open up, lengthening your legs and lowering your torso back to the starting position.

4 Repeat the motion without completely lying down on the mat. Repeat 15 times for two sets.

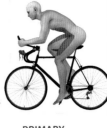

PRIMARY TARGETS
- rectus abdominis
- obliquus internus
- obliquus externus
- transversus abdominis
- tensor fasciae latae
- vastus intermedius
- rectus femoris
- vastus medialis
- piriformis

BENEFITS
- Increases abdominal endurance
- Strengthens hip flexors

CAUTIONS
- Lower-back pain

PERFECT YOUR FORM
- Keep your chin tucked.
- Keep your thighs firm throughout the exercise.
- Avoid allowing your shoulders to lift up toward your ears.

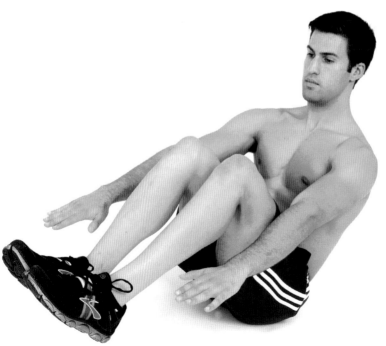

BUILDING CORE STRENGTH & STABILITY

ABDOMINAL HIP LIFT

INTERMEDIATE

ANOTHER POWERFUL ABDOMINAL TONER to add to your cycling workout is the Abdominal Hip Lift. It specifically targets the rectus abdominis (the long "six-pack" muscle running between your ribs and hips) and the obliques (the external and internal muscles that run down the sides of your torso).

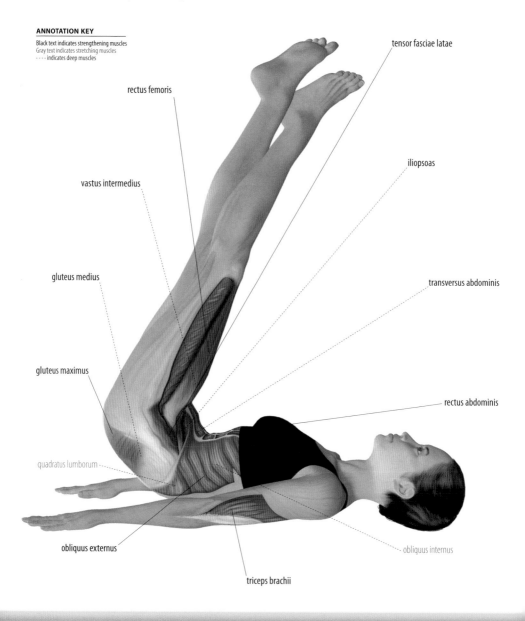

ANNOTATION KEY
Black text indicates strengthening muscles
Gray text indicates stretching muscles
- - - - indicates deep muscles

tensor fasciae latae

rectus femoris

iliopsoas

vastus intermedius

transversus abdominis

gluteus medius

gluteus maximus

rectus abdominis

quadratus lumborum

obliquus externus

obliquus internus

triceps brachii

HOW TO DO IT

1 Lie down with your legs in the air and crossed at the ankles, knees straight. Place your arms on the floor, straight by your sides.

2 Pinching your legs together and squeezing your buttocks, press into the back of your arms to lift your hips upward.

3 Slowly return your hips to the floor. Repeat 10 times, and then switch with the opposite leg crossed in the front.

For a greater challenge, keep your hips on the floor, and raise your arms toward the ceiling. Reach toward your toes as you lift your shoulders off the floor.

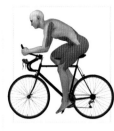

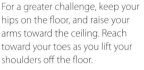

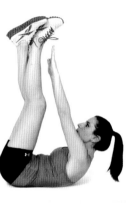

PRIMARY TARGETS
- rectus abdominis
- transversus abdominis
- vastus intermedius
- tensor fasciae latae
- gluteus maximus
- gluteus medius
- triceps brachii
- rectus femoris
- iliopsoas

BENEFITS
- Strengthens core and pelvic stabilizers
- Firms and tones lower abdominals

CAUTIONS
- Back pain
- Neck pain
- Shoulder pain

PERFECT YOUR FORM
- Keep your legs straight and firm throughout the exercise.
- Relax your neck and shoulders as you lift your hips.
- Keep all of your movements smooth.
- Avoid using momentum to lift your hips.

ABDOMINAL KICK

INTERMEDIATE

THE ABDOMINAL KICK stabilizes your entire core and strengthens your abdominal muscles, especially your transversus abdominis, or lower abs. This exercise trains you to move from your center, using your abdominal muscles to initiate movement and to support and stabilize your trunk as your arms and legs are in motion. It can also help improve your overall coordination.

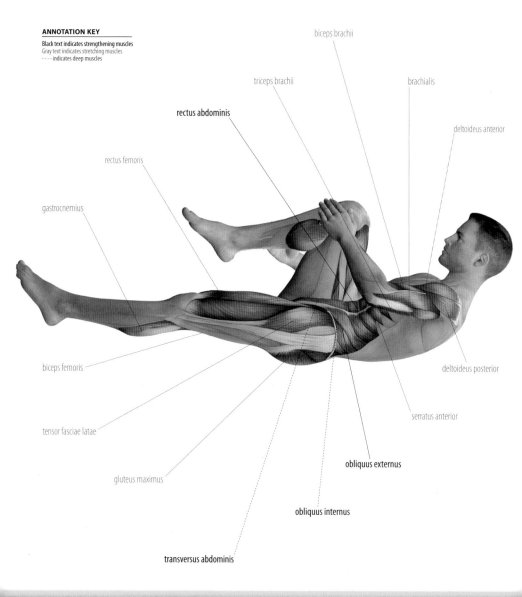

ANNOTATION KEY

Black text indicates strengthening muscles
Gray text indicates stretching muscles
- - - - indicates deep muscles

biceps brachii

triceps brachii

brachialis

rectus abdominis

deltoideus anterior

rectus femoris

gastrocnemius

deltoideus posterior

biceps femoris

serratus anterior

tensor fasciae latae

obliquus externus

gluteus maximus

obliquus internus

transversus abdominis

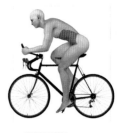

HOW TO DO IT

1 Lie on your back with your legs extended. Pull your right knee toward your chest and straighten your left leg, raising it 45 degrees from the floor.

2 Place your right hand on your right ankle and your left hand on your right knee to maintain proper leg alignment.

3 Switch your legs two times, switching your hand placement simultaneously.

4 Switch your legs two more times, keeping your hands in their proper placement. Repeat four to six times.

PRIMARY TARGETS
- rectus abdominis
- transversus abdominis
- obliquus externus
- obliquus internus

BENEFITS
- Stabilizes core while extremities are in motion
- Strengthens abdominals

CAUTIONS
- Neck issues
- Lower-back pain

PERFECT YOUR FORM
- Place your outside hand on the ankle of your bent leg and your inside hand on your bent knee.
- Lift your chest.
- Avoid allowing your lower back to rise off the floor; use your abdominals to stabilize your core while switching legs.

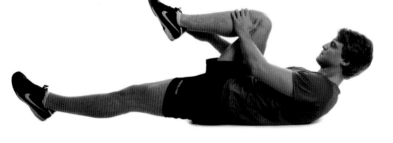

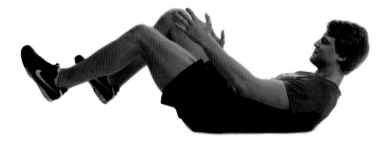

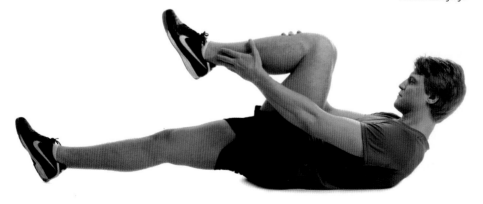

BRIDGE WITH LEG LIFT

INTERMEDIATE

THE BRIDGE WITH LEG LIFT efficiently strengthens your abdominals, gluteals, and hamstrings while adding a workout for your hip flexors—the rectus femoris, iliopsoas, and sartorius muscles. The hip flexors allow you to perform the basic cycling moves of lifting your knees and bending at the waist.

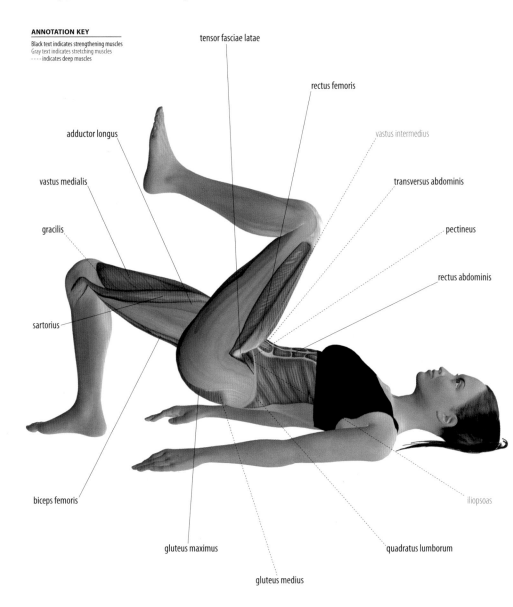

ANNOTATION KEY

Black text indicates strengthening muscles
Gray text indicates stretching muscles
---- indicates deep muscles

tensor fasciae latae

rectus femoris

adductor longus

vastus intermedius

vastus medialis

transversus abdominis

gracilis

pectineus

rectus abdominis

sartorius

biceps femoris

iliopsoas

gluteus maximus

quadratus lumborum

gluteus medius

HOW TO DO IT

1 Lie in supine position on the floor, your arms by your sides and lengthened toward your feet. Your legs should be bent with your feet flat on the floor.

2 Lift your hips and spine off the floor, creating one long line from your knees to your shoulders. Keep your weight shifted over your feet.

3 Keeping your legs bent, bring your left knee toward your chest.

4 Lower your left leg until your toe touches the mat. Be sure to keep your pelvis level.

5 Bring your left knee toward your chest again. Repeat entire sequence four to five times.

6 Lower your left leg to the floor, switch legs, and repeat the exercise with your right leg. Repeat entire sequence four to five times.

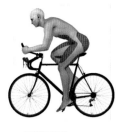

PRIMARY TARGETS
- rectus abdominis
- transversus abdominis
- quadratus lumborum
- gluteus medius
- gluteus maximus
- biceps femoris
- iliopsoas
- rectus femoris
- sartorius
- tensor fasciae latae
- pectineus
- adductor longus
- gracilis

BENEFITS
- Improves pelvic and spinal stability
- Increases hip flexor endurance

CAUTIONS
- Neck issues
- Knee injury

PERFECT YOUR FORM
- To keep your hips and torso stable, you can prop yourself up with your hands beneath your hips once you are in the bridge position.
- Tightly squeeze your glutes as you scoop in your abdominals for stability.
- Avoid extending out of your hip, which allows your back to do the work.
- Avoid lifting your hips so high that your weight shifts onto your neck.

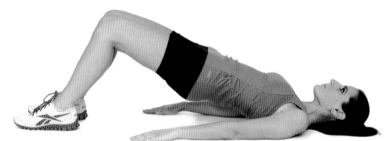

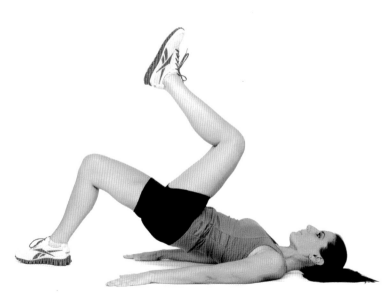

SIDE-BEND PLANK

INTERMEDIATE

THE SIDE BEND PLANK, with its Pilates pedigree, is a powerful core strengthener that also increases spine flexibility. Look to keep your spine straight and even from shoulder to hip to efficiently transfer weight from your arms and upper body and avoid excessive strain on your shoulder girdle.

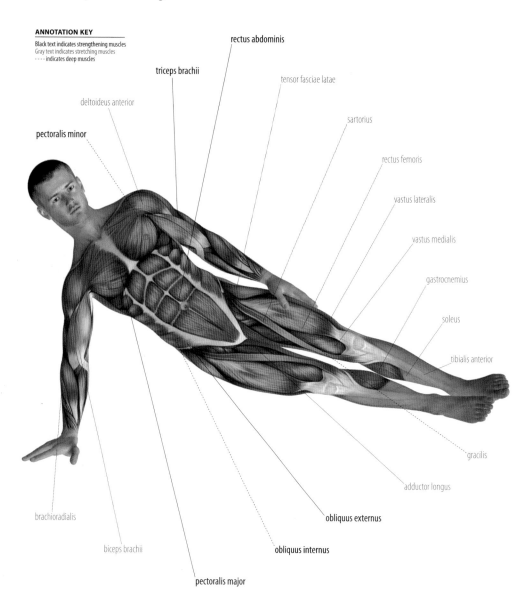

ANNOTATION KEY

Black text indicates strengthening muscles
Gray text indicates stretching muscles
---- indicates deep muscles

rectus abdominis

triceps brachii

tensor fasciae latae

deltoideus anterior

sartorius

pectoralis minor

rectus femoris

vastus lateralis

vastus medialis

gastrocnemius

soleus

tibialis anterior

gracilis

adductor longus

brachioradialis

obliquus externus

biceps brachii

obliquus internus

pectoralis major

HOW TO DO IT

1 Lie on your right side with one arm supporting your torso, aligning your wrist under your shoulder. Place your left arm on top of your left leg, and strongly squeeze them together in adduction with legs parallel and feet flexed. Draw your navel toward your spine.

2 Press downward into the palm of your right hand, and lift your hips off the floor, creating a straight line between your heels and head.

3 Slowly lower your hips, returning to the starting position. Repeat sequence five to six times, keeping your legs tight and your glutes squeezed. Repeat the sequence on the other side.

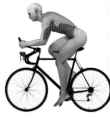

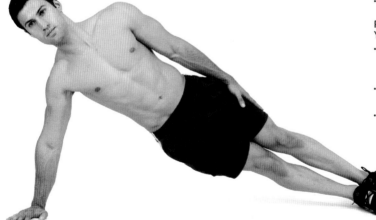

BUILDING CORE STRENGTH & STABILITY

PRIMARY TARGETS
• rectus abdominis
• obliquus internus
• obliquus externus
• adductor magnus
• pectoralis major
• pectoralis minor
• triceps brachii
• gluteus medius

BENEFITS
• Stabilizes spine in neutral position with the support of shoulder girdle

CAUTIONS
• Rotator cuff injury
• Neck issues

PERFECT YOUR FORM
• Lift your hips high to take some weight off your upper body.
• Elongate your limbs as much as possible.
• Avoid allowing your shoulders to sink into their sockets or lift toward your ears.

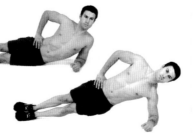

Beginners can try this easier version of the Side-Bend Plank. Rather than supporting your torso with your arm straight, bend your elbow so that it is aligned below your shoulder. Press into your forearm to lift your body into the side plank position.

FRONT PLANK EXTENSION

ADVANCED

PACKING A POWERFUL PUNCH, the Front Plank Extension targets your leg, abdominal, shoulder, and arm muscles. This exercise calls for you to maintain a stable position while achieving full-body extension and flexion.

ANNOTATION KEY
Black text indicates strengthening muscles
Gray text indicates stretching muscles
- - - - indicates deep muscles

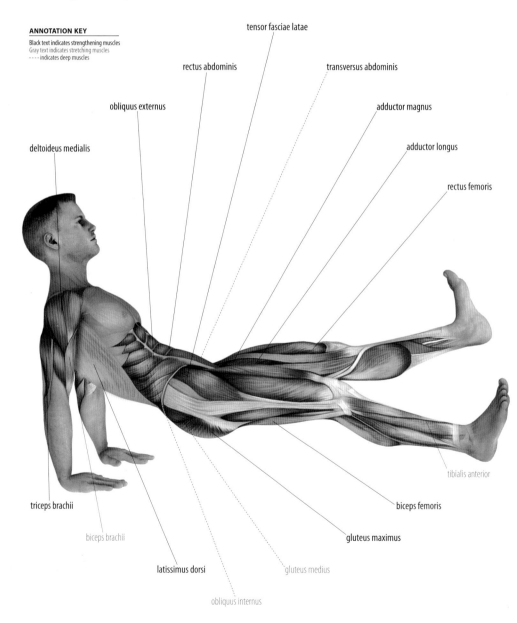

tensor fasciae latae

rectus abdominis

transversus abdominis

obliquus externus

adductor magnus

deltoideus medialis

adductor longus

rectus femoris

triceps brachii

tibialis anterior

biceps brachii

biceps femoris

gluteus maximus

latissimus dorsi

gluteus medius

obliquus internus

HOW TO DO IT

1 Sit with your legs parallel and extended out in front of you. Place your hands behind you with your fingers pointed toward your hips.

2 Press up through your arms and lift your chest up, squeezing your glutes and lifting your hips while pressing your heels into the floor. Continue lifting your pelvis until your body forms a long line from your shoulders to your feet.

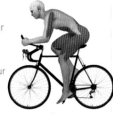

3 Without allowing your pelvis to drop, keep your left leg straight, and raise it as high as you comfortably can.

4 Slowly lower your left leg to the floor, and switch to the right leg. Repeat four to six times on each side.

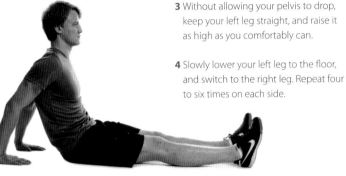

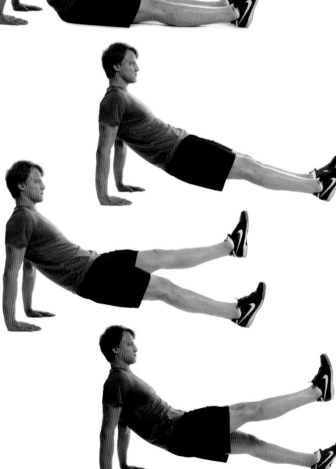

PRIMARY TARGETS
- rectus abdominis
- transversus abdominis
- gluteus maximus
- biceps femoris
- deltoideus
- rectus femoris
- adductor magnus
- tensor fasciae latae
- adductor longus
- obliquus externus
- latissimus dorsi
- triceps brachii

BENEFITS
- Strengthens core muscles and deep stabilizing muscles

CAUTIONS
- Wrist pain
- Knee pain
- Shoulder injury
- Shooting pains down leg

PERFECT YOUR FORM
- Elevate your pelvis throughout the exercise.
- Avoid allowing your shoulders to sink into their sockets.
- If your legs do not feel strong enough to support your body, slightly bend your knees.

BUILDING CORE STRENGTH & STABILITY

V-UP

ADVANCED

TAKE YOUR CORE WORKOUT to another level with the challenging V-Up. This exercise targets the rectus abdominis while working your quadriceps and lower-back muscles. Performing the full movement also increases spinal flexibility and range of motion.

ANNOTATION KEY

Black text indicates strengthening muscles
Gray text indicates stretching muscles
- - - - indicates deep muscles

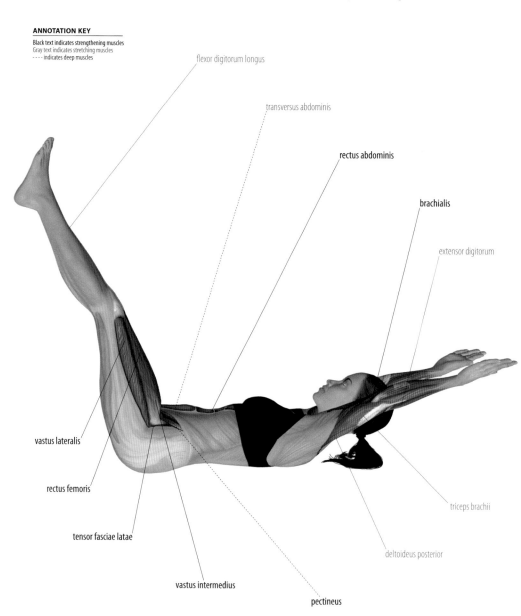

flexor digitorum longus

transversus abdominis

rectus abdominis

brachialis

extensor digitorum

vastus lateralis

rectus femoris

tensor fasciae latae

vastus intermedius

pectineus

triceps brachii

deltoideus posterior

HOW TO DO IT

1 Lie on your back with your legs raised at an angle between 45 and 90 degrees.

2 Inhale, reaching your arms toward the ceiling as you lift your head and shoulders off the floor.

3 Exhale, and while rolling through your spine, lift your rib cage off the floor to just before the sit bones.

4 Inhale, and reach your arms toward your toes while maintaining a C curve in your back. Exhale, and roll down your spine by articulating one vertebra at a time. Return to the starting position.

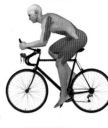

PRIMARY TARGETS
- rectus abdominis
- tensor fasciae latae
- rectus femoris
- vastus lateralis
- vastus medialis
- vastus intermedius
- adductor longus
- pectineus
- brachialis

BENEFITS
- Strengthens abdominals while mobilizing the spine

CAUTIONS
- Advanced osteoporosis
- A herniated disc
- Lower-back pain

PERFECT YOUR FORM
- Articulate through your spine on the way up and on the way down.
- Keep your neck elongated and relaxed, minimizing the tension in your upper spine.
- Avoid using momentum to carry you through the exercise; use your abdominal muscles to lift your legs and torso.

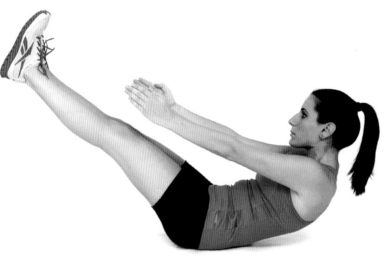

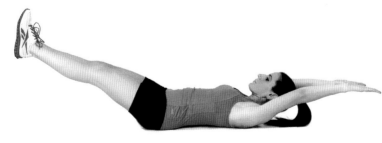

FOAM ROLLER DEAD BUG

ADVANCED

TAKING ITS NAME from the legs-up position of a dead beetle, the Dead Bug is a great exercise for working both your upper and lower abdominals. Performing this move on a mat is relatively simple, but adding the foam roller injects an element of instability that forces you to fully engage your abs. Foam Roller Dead Bug also improves arm and leg coordination and your sense of balance.

ANNOTATION KEY

Black text indicates strengthening muscles
Gray text indicates stretching muscles
- - - - indicates deep muscles

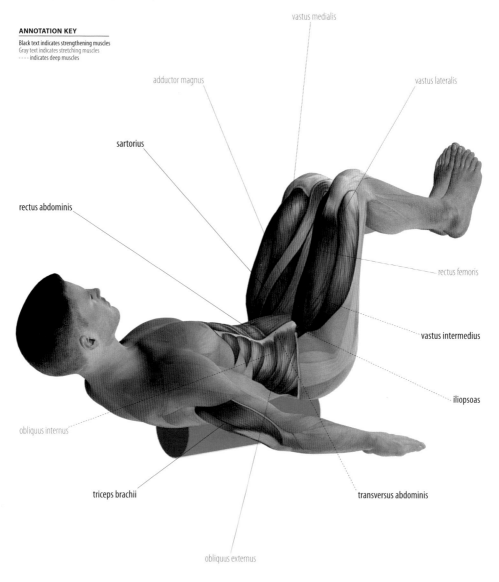

vastus medialis

adductor magnus

vastus lateralis

sartorius

rectus abdominis

rectus femoris

vastus intermedius

iliopsoas

obliquus internus

triceps brachii

transversus abdominis

obliquus externus

HOW TO DO IT

1 Lie on your back with a foam roller placed lengthwise under your spine, your buttocks and shoulders resting on the roller. Place your hands and forearms flat on the floor for stabilization. Draw your knees up so that your legs form a tabletop position.

2 Lift your head, neck, and shoulders.

3 Press the palms of your hands onto your knees, creating your own resistance as you try to balance. Flex your toes and keep your elbows pulled in to your sides. Hold for 10 seconds. Repeat 10 times.

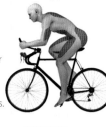

PRIMARY TARGETS
- rectus abdominis
- transversus abdominis
- gluteus maximus
- gluteus medius
- sartorius
- vastus intermedius
- iliopsoas
- infraspinatus
- supraspinatus
- teres minor
- erector spinae
- triceps brachii

BENEFITS
- Improves pelvic and core stabilization
- Strengthens abdominals

CAUTIONS
- Lower-back pain
- Neck pain

PERFECT YOUR FORM
- Look for your hips, thighs, and calves to form a 90-degree angle.
- Keep your neck relaxed throughout the exercise.
- Keep your shoulders and buttocks flat on the roller.
- Avoid hunching your shoulders.
- Avoid lifting your hips or lower back during the movement.

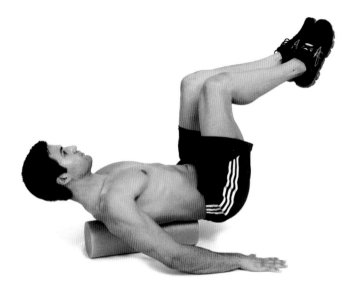

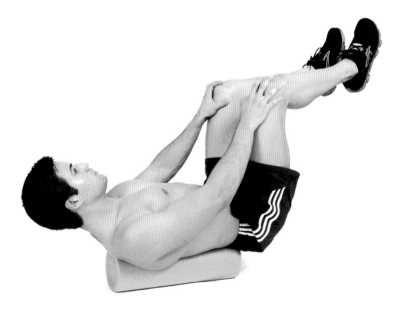

FOAM ROLLER BICYCLE

ADVANCED

ANOTHER RELATIVELY SIMPLY EXERCISE when performed on a mat, the Bicycle mimics the pedaling motion of cycling, engaging your core and increasing pelvic stability. Performing this exercise on a foam roller boosts it to another level—you must fully engage your abdominals in order to stay in place atop the roller.

ANNOTATION KEY
Black text indicates strengthening muscles
Gray text indicates stretching muscles
- - - - indicates deep muscles

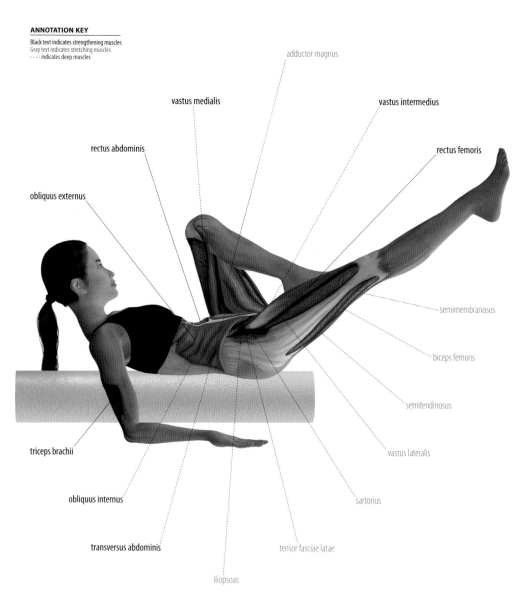

adductor magnus

vastus medialis

vastus intermedius

rectus abdominis

rectus femoris

obliquus externus

semimembranosus

biceps femoris

semitendinosus

triceps brachii

vastus lateralis

obliquus internus

sartorius

transversus abdominis

tensor fasciae latae

iliopsoas

HOW TO DO IT

1 Lie on your back with a foam roller placed lengthwise under your spine, your buttocks and shoulders resting on the roller. Place your forearms on the floor on either side of the roller to balance yourself.

2 Draw your knees up to a tabletop position, forming a 90-degree angle between your hips, thighs, and calves.

3 Keeping your back flat, lift your head, neck, and shoulders off the roller. Straighten your right leg and pull your left knee in toward your chest, keeping your head, neck, and shoulders lifted.

4 Switch legs while maintaining your balance, imitating the pedalling of a bike. Repeat 15 times on each leg.

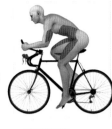

PRIMARY TARGETS
- rectus abdominis
- transversus abdominis
- obliquus internus
- obliquus externus
- triceps brachii
- vastus intermedius
- rectus femoris
- vastus medialis

BENEFITS
- Improves pelvic stabilization
- Strengthens abdominals

CAUTIONS
- Lower-back pain
- Neck pain

PERFECT YOUR FORM
LOOK FOR
- Keep your neck relaxed throughout the exercise.
- Fully extend your leg during the downward phase of the "pedaling" movement.
- Avoid allowing your shoulders to lift toward your ears.
- Avoid lifting your hips and lower back during the movement.

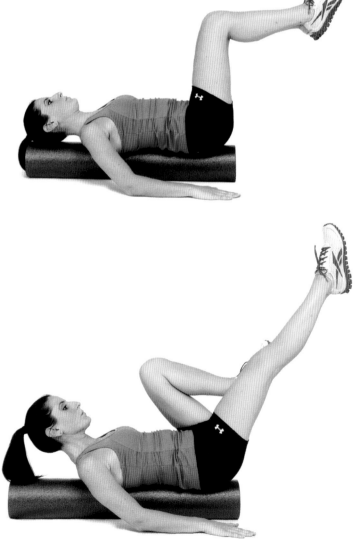

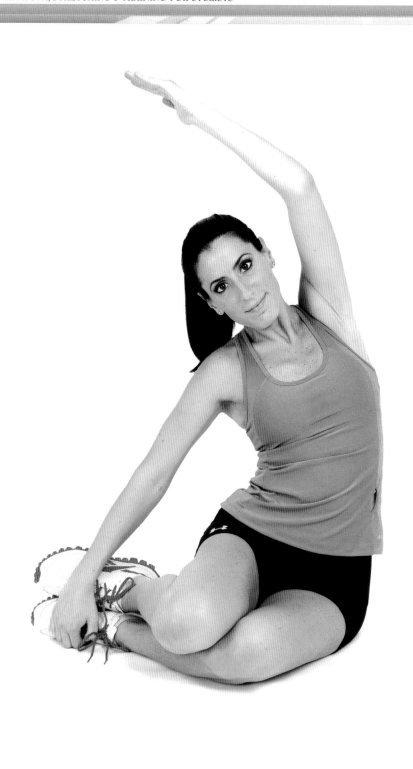

IMPROVING YOUR POSTURE, BALANCE & COORDINATION

Riding a bicycle is all about balance, so cyclists should work on improving theirs. Exercises that improve balance and posture will enhance the positive effects of your strengthening, stretching, and stabilizing moves. These exercises bring multiple parts of the body into play; the goal is harmonious movement that comes from a solid center.

After all, cyclists need to consider so much more than developing leg strength. Many of the exercises that follow will build back strength and stability. An exercise like Swimming, for instance, counterbalances forward flexion movements and is essential in counteracting the effects of sitting forward on your bike, holding handlebars for hours on end. And Rolling Like a Ball works the abdominal muscles evenly as it deeply releases and massages the lower back, which so often troubles cyclists. Be patient as you explore these exercises. Over time, you will build a balance and posture regimen that works for you.

QUADRUPED LEG LIFT

BEGINNER

CONNECTING YOUR ARMS and legs with your core while focusing on balancing and stability is a key goal of the Quadruped Leg Lift. This exercise helps tone all the muscles along the body's central axis in one powerful, extending movement.

ANNOTATION KEY

Black text indicates strengthening muscles
Gray text indicates stretching muscles
- - - - indicates deep muscles

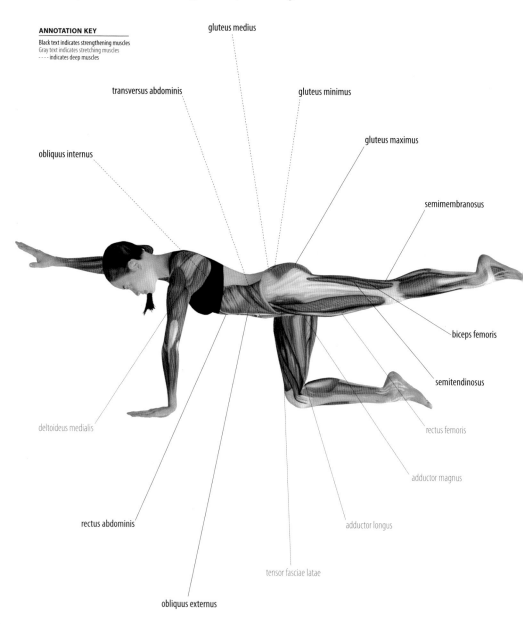

gluteus medius

transversus abdominis

gluteus minimus

obliquus internus

gluteus maximus

semimembranosus

biceps femoris

semitendinosus

deltoideus medialis

rectus femoris

adductor magnus

rectus abdominis

adductor longus

tensor fasciae latae

obliquus externus

HOW TO DO IT

1 Kneeling on all fours, connect with your abdominals by drawing your navel up toward your spine.

2 Slowly raise your right arm and extend your left leg, all while keeping your torso still. Extend your arm and leg until they are both parallel to the floor, creating one long line with your body. Do not allow your pelvis to bend or rotate.

3 Bring your arm and leg back into the starting position.

4 Repeat sequence on the other side, alternating sides six times.

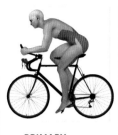

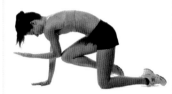

This variation will give your abs a greater challenge. Follow steps 1 and 2, and then draw your opposite knee and elbow inward to touch. Repeat entire sequence on the other side.

PRIMARY TARGETS
- rectus abdominis
- transversus abdominis
- obliquus internus
- obliquus externus
- gluteus maximus
- gluteus minimus
- gluteus medius
- biceps femoris
- semitendinosus
- semimembranosus

BENEFITS
- Tones arms, legs, and abdominals

CAUTIONS
- Wrist pain
- Lower-back pain
- Knee pain
- Inability to stabilize the spine while moving limbs

PERFECT YOUR FORM
- Move slowly and steadily to decrease pelvic rotation.
- Engage your abs by drawing your navel toward your spine.

IMPROVING YOUR POSTURE, BALANCE & COORDINATION

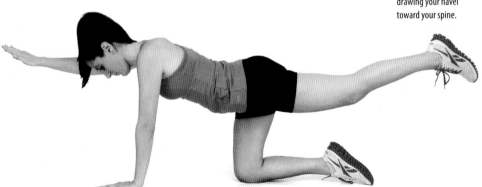

SWIMMING

BEGINNER

SWIMMING IS A FUN EXERCISE that calls on the same muscles that you use while swimming. Without stepping into a pool, you will engage just about every muscle in your body. Use your exercise mat for stability, and aim for a long, full stretch in you arms and legs. As your head and shoulders come up off the mat, let your spine lengthen as well.

ANNOTATION KEY
Black text indicates strengthening muscles
Gray text indicates stretching muscles
- - - - indicates deep muscles

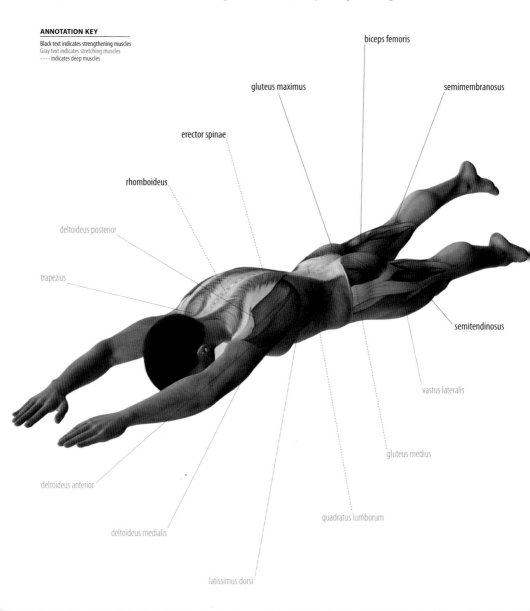

biceps femoris

gluteus maximus

semimembranosus

erector spinae

rhomboideus

deltoideus posterior

trapezius

semitendinosus

vastus lateralis

deltoideus anterior

gluteus medius

deltoideus medialis

quadratus lumborum

latissimus dorsi

HOW TO DO IT

1 Lie prone on the floor with your legs hip-width apart. Stretch your arms beside your ears on the floor. Engage your pelvic floor, and draw your navel toward your spine.

2 Extend through your upper back as you lift your left arm and right leg simultaneously. Lift your head and shoulders off the floor.

3 Lower your arm and leg to the starting position, maintaining a stretch in your limbs throughout.

4 Extend your right arm and left leg off the floor, lengthening and lifting your head and shoulders.

5 Elongate your limbs as you return to the starting position. Repeat six to eight times.

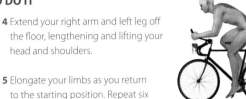

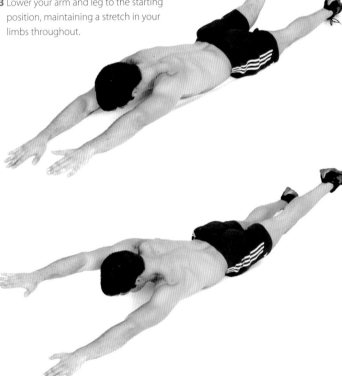

To add a challenge to this exercise, instead of lifting the opposite leg and arm, lift both arms and legs simultaneously, continuing to draw your navel into your spine. This version of the exercise is commonly known as the Superman.

PRIMARY TARGETS
- gluteus maximus
- biceps femoris
- semitendinosus
- semimembranosus
- erector spinae
- rhomboideus

BENEFITS
- Strengthens hip and spine extensors
- Challenges stabilization of the spine against rotation
- Improves coordination

CAUTIONS
- Lower-back pain
- Extreme curvature of the upper spine
- Curvature of the lower spine

PERFECT YOUR FORM
- Extend your limbs as far as possible in opposite directions.
- Squeeze your glutes and draw your navel into your spine throughout.
- Keep your neck elongated and relaxed.
- Avoid allowing your shoulders to lift toward your ears.

IMPROVING YOUR POSTURE, BALANCE & COORDINATION

ROLLING LIKE A BALL

BEGINNER

ONE OF THE PILATES CLASSICAL EXERCISES, Rolling Like a Ball, demands balance and control while it articulates and stretches your spine. A great exercise to help you to develop core control, it also gives your back a soothing massage.

ANNOTATION KEY

Black text indicates strengthening muscles
Gray text indicates stretching muscles
- - - - indicates deep muscles

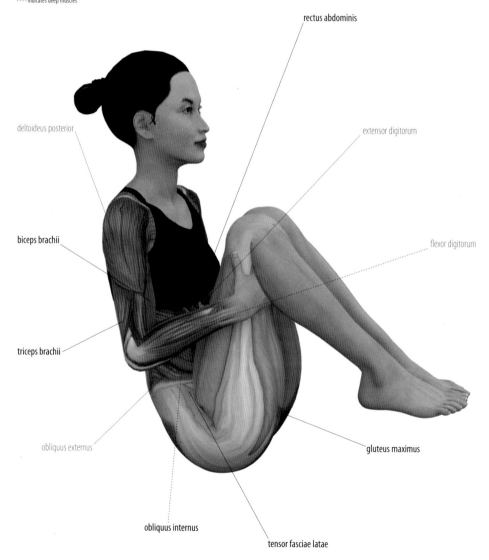

rectus abdominis

deltoideus posterior

extensor digitorum

biceps brachii

flexor digitorum

triceps brachii

obliquus externus

gluteus maximus

obliquus internus

tensor fasciae latae

HOW TO DO IT

1 Sitting with your legs bent and feet raised off the floor, find your balance point. Place your hands around the backs of your thighs.

2 Using your lower abdominals to lift your hips, roll back onto your shoulders.

3 Exhale, and using your abdominal muscles, roll up to your balancing point. Keep your shoulders relaxed throughout the movement.

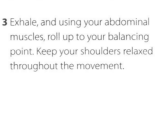

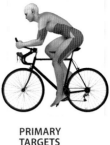

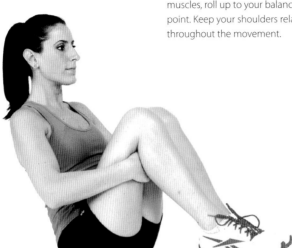

PRIMARY TARGETS
- rectus abdominis
- triceps brachii
- biceps brachii
- gluteus maximus
- tensor fasciae latae
- transversus abdominis
- obliquus internus

BENEFITS
- Improves balance and coordination
- Massages back muscles
- Enhances core and abdominal control

CAUTIONS
- Neck issues

PERFECT YOUR FORM
- Look for your back to curve throughout the movement.
- Use your abdominal muscles to maintain your balance.
- Avoid using your arm muscles to roll and balance your body.
- Avoid allowing your feet to touch the ground.

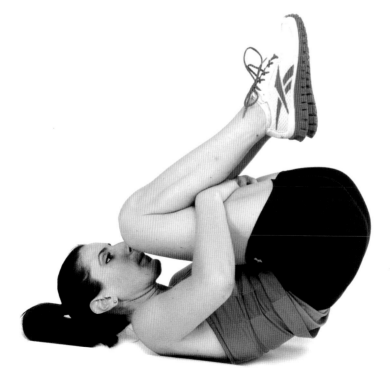

IMPROVING YOUR POSTURE, BALANCE & COORDINATION

KNEE SQUAT

BEGINNER

THE KNEE SQUAT integrates balance, coordination, resistance, and stretching to target your leg muscles. This exercise also strengthens the muscles of your feet.

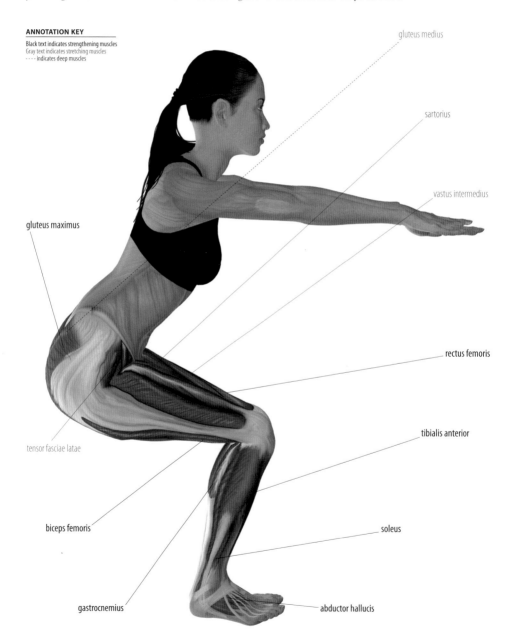

ANNOTATION KEY
Black text indicates strengthening muscles
Gray text indicates stretching muscles
- - - - indicates deep muscles

gluteus medius

sartorius

vastus intermedius

gluteus maximus

rectus femoris

tensor fasciae latae

tibialis anterior

biceps femoris

soleus

gastrocnemius

abductor hallucis

HOW TO DO IT

1 Stand with your legs and feet parallel and shoulder-width apart, and your knees bent very slightly. Tuck your pelvis slightly forward, lift your chest, and press your shoulders downward and back.

2 Extend your arms in front of your body for stability, keeping them even with your shoulders. Plant your feet firmly on the floor, and curl your toes slightly upward.

3 Draw in your abdominal muscles and bend into a squat. Keep your heels planted on the floor and your chest as upright as possible, resisting the urge to bend too far forward.

4 Exhale, and return to the original position. Repeat five to six times.

PRIMARY TARGETS
- biceps femoris
- rectus femoris
- tibialis anterior
- gastrocnemius
- soleus
- gluteus maximus
- abductor hallucis
- vastus medialis

BENEFITS
- Improves balance
- Lengthens and strengthens calf muscles

CAUTIONS
- Foot pain

PERFECT YOUR FORM
- Keep your chest upright.
- Pull your abdominals in toward your spine.
- Curl your toes upward throughout the movement.
- Imagine pressing into the floor as you rise from the squat, creating your body's own resistance in your leg muscles.
- Avoid allowing your heels to lift off the floor.
- Avoid rising too quickly to the standing position.

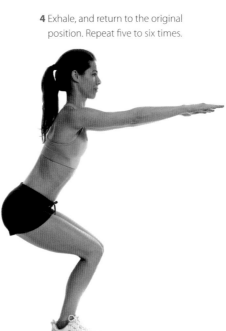

Challenge yourself by adding weight to this exercise by grasping a weighted medicine ball in both hands, and then following steps 1 though 4.

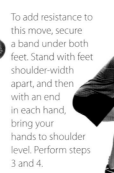

To add resistance to this move, secure a band under both feet. Stand with feet shoulder-width apart, and then with an end in each hand, bring your hands to shoulder level. Perform steps 3 and 4.

SIDE MERMAID

INTERMEDIATE

THE SIDE MERMAID IS AN INVIGORATING EXERCISE that gives your upper body a complete stretch. It can improve your posture by helping you to maintain a healthy and supple spine. It will also lengthen and strengthen your obliques, the layers of external and internal muscles running along the sides of your torso that shape your waistline. The Side Mermaid helps eliminate "love handles" and "spare tires"—those excess bulges you may be carrying around your midsection.

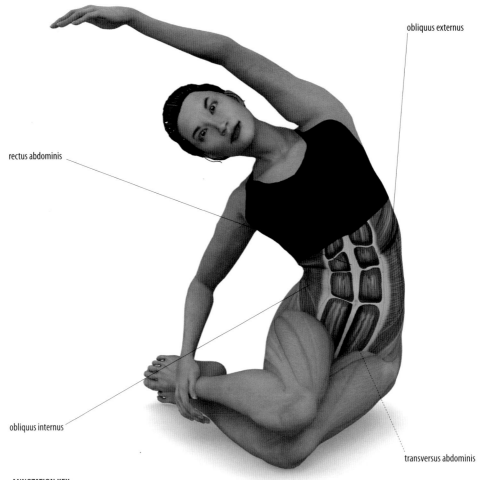

obliquus externus

rectus abdominis

obliquus internus

transversus abdominis

ANNOTATION KEY

Black text indicates strengthening muscles
Gray text indicates stretching muscles
- - - - indicates deep muscles

HOW TO DO IT

1 Sit with your knees bent and your right leg folded on top of your left leg. Place your right hand on your right ankle or foot. Inhale, reaching your left arm toward the ceiling.

2 Exhale, reaching your left arm in the direction of your ankles, pulling your navel toward your spine and rotating the torso slightly backward.

3 Inhale, and then return to the starting position. Switch legs, and repeat on the other side.

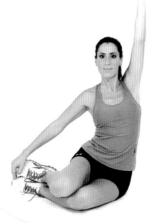

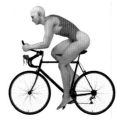

PRIMARY TARGETS
• rectus abdominis
• transversus abdominis
• obliquus internus
• obliquus externus
• latissimus dorsi

BENEFITS
• Stretches spine and entire torso
• Opens up chest and tight back muscles

CAUTIONS
• Intense back pain
• Hip pain rooted deeply in the joints

PERFECT YOUR FORM
• Reach your arm as far as you can to open your chest and reach a maximum stretch.
• If you experience knee pain while in the initial position, sit on a pillow or straighten your top leg to the side.

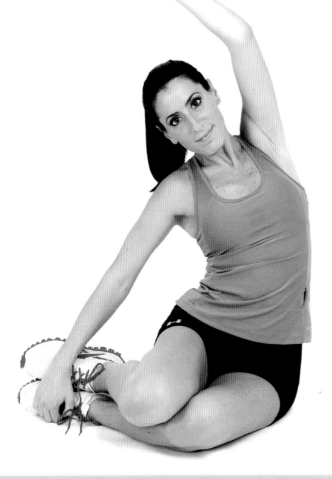

IMPROVING YOUR POSTURE, BALANCE & COORDINATION

STANDING KNEE CRUNCH

INTERMEDIATE

THE STANDING KNEE CRUNCH has all the benefits of a Basic Crunch—strengthening your abdominals—while also challenging your coordination and sense of balance.

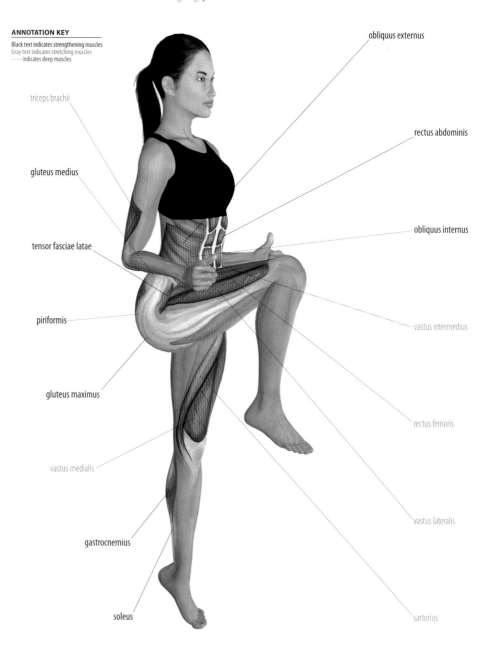

ANNOTATION KEY
Black text indicates strengthening muscles
Gray text indicates stretching muscles
---- indicates deep muscles

triceps brachii

gluteus medius

tensor fasciae latae

piriformis

gluteus maximus

vastus medialis

gastrocnemius

soleus

obliquus externus

rectus abdominis

obliquus internus

vastus intermedius

rectus femoris

vastus lateralis

sartorius

HOW TO DO IT

1 Stand tall with your left leg in front of the right, and extend your hands toward the ceiling, your arms straight.

2 Shift your weight onto your left foot, and raise your right knee to the height of your hips. To create the crunch, simultaneously lift up on the toes of your left leg while pulling your elbows down by your sides, your hands making fists.

3 Pause at the top of the movement, and then return to the starting position. Repeat the sequence with your right leg as the standing leg. Repeat 10 times on each leg.

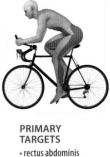

PRIMARY TARGETS
- rectus abdominis
- obliquus internus
- obliquus externus
- transversus abdominis
- gluteus maximus
- gluteus medius
- tensor fasciae latae
- piriformis
- iliopsoas
- gastrocnemius
- soleus

BENEFITS
- Strengthens core
- Strengthens calves and gluteal muscles
- Improves balance

CAUTIONS
- Knee pain

PERFECT YOUR FORM
- Keep your standing leg straight as you rise up on your toes.
- Relax your shoulders as you pull your arms down for the crunch.
- Flex the toes of your raised leg.
- Avoid tilting forward as you switch legs.

IMPROVING YOUR POSTURE, BALANCE & COORDINATION

OPEN-LEG ROCKER

ADVANCED

THE OPEN-LEG ROCKER is a low-intensity Pilates exercise that strengthens the muscles of your back and abdominals while helping you to develop your sense of balance and coordination. As you perform the rocking motion of this exercise, be sure to fully engage your core and use your arms to maintain your balance.

ANNOTATION KEY

Black text indicates strengthening muscles
Gray text indicates stretching muscles
- - - - indicates deep muscles

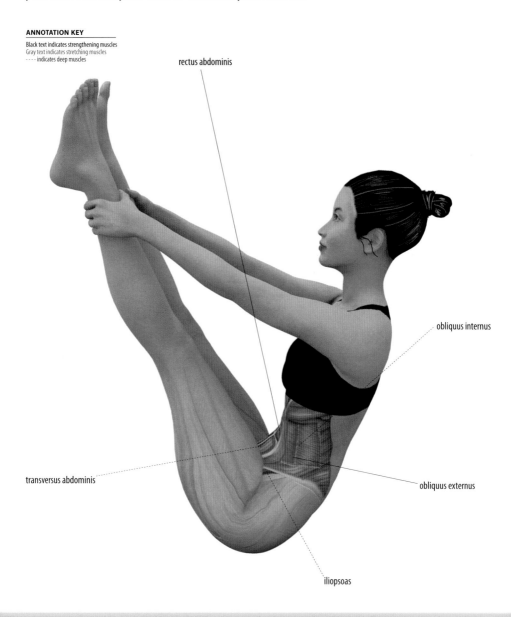

rectus abdominis

obliquus internus

transversus abdominis

obliquus externus

iliopsoas

HOW TO DO IT

1 Sitting on a mat, lift your legs and grasp your ankles or calves. Your legs should be abducted and parallel with your knees straight.

2 Inhale, scooping your abdominals in while rolling off your sit bones until your legs are parallel to the floor. Do not allow your weight to extend beyond mid scapula.

3 Exhale, rolling your body back to the starting position. Repeat six to eight times.

PRIMARY TARGETS
• rectus abdominis
• obliquus internus
• obliquus externus
• transversus abdominis
• iliopsoas

BENEFITS
• Develops stability in the spine through the rocking motion

CAUTIONS
• A herniated disc

PERFECT YOUR FORM
• Deeply scoop your abdominals.
• Keep your neck elongated and relaxed.
• Avoid rolling back onto your neck. If you have trouble stopping, bend your knees slightly as you return to the starting position.

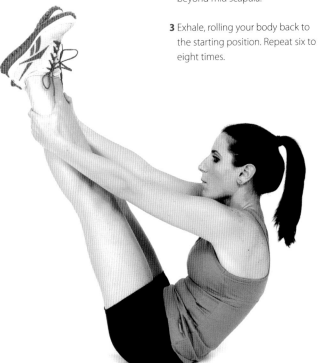

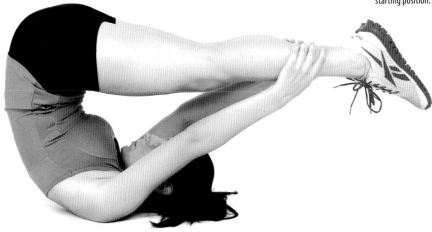

IMPROVING YOUR POSTURE, BALANCE & COORDINATION

THREE-LEGGED DOG

ADVANCED

THIS EXERCISE IS A VARIATION of the traditional Downward-Facing Dog posture of yoga, which calls for you to balance on all four limbs to strengthen your arm and leg muscles and create space in your torso for better organ function. Three-Legged Dog adds a further challenge by adding a backward leg extension to an asymmetrical balance.

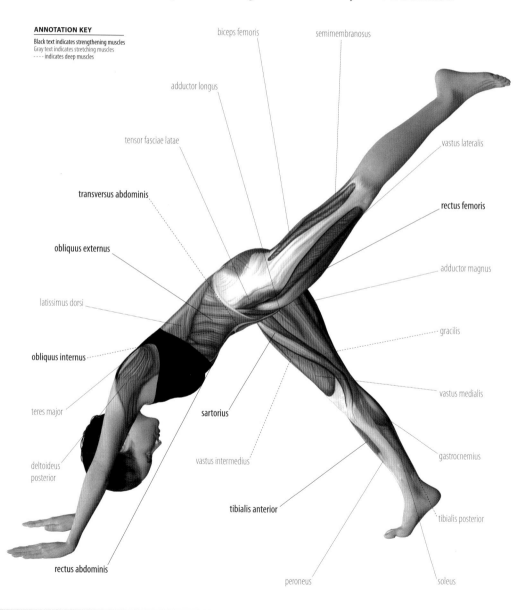

ANNOTATION KEY

Black text indicates strengthening muscles
Gray text indicates stretching muscles
---- indicates deep muscles

biceps femoris

semimembranosus

adductor longus

tensor fasciae latae

vastus lateralis

transversus abdominis

rectus femoris

obliquus externus

adductor magnus

latissimus dorsi

gracilis

obliquus internus

vastus medialis

teres major

sartorius

deltoideus posterior

vastus intermedius

gastrocnemius

tibialis posterior

tibialis anterior

rectus abdominis

peroneus

soleus

HOW TO DO IT

1 Start in plank position with your shoulders directly over your hands, your torso straight, and your weight distributed evenly between your arms and legs.

2 Draw your left knee into your chest, flexing your foot while rocking your body forward over your hands. You should come up on the toes of your right foot.

3 Extend your left knee backward, rocking your body back, and shifting your weight onto your heel. With your head in between your hands, straighten your right leg and lift it toward the ceiling. Repeat 10 times on each leg.

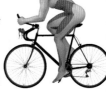

PRIMARY TARGETS
- rectus abdominis
- transversus abdominis
- sartorius
- obliquus externus
- obliquus internus
- rectus femoris
- tibialis anterior

BENEFITS
- Stabilizes core
- Stabilizes shoulders
- Stretches calves and hamstrings

CAUTIONS
- Sharp lower-back pain
- Wrist pain
- Ankle pain

PERFECT YOUR FORM
- Align your shoulders over your hands.
- Flex your toes inward during the movement.
- Avoid bending the knee of the supporting leg.

SIDE PLANK BALANCE

ADVANCED

THE SIDE PLANK BALANCE exercise, also known as T-Stabilization, is a challenging variation of the traditional plank. It targets your abdominals, hips, lower back, and obliques while also helping you to improve your sense of balance and stability.

ANNOTATION KEY

Black text indicates strengthening muscles
Gray text indicates stretching muscles
- - - - indicates deep muscles

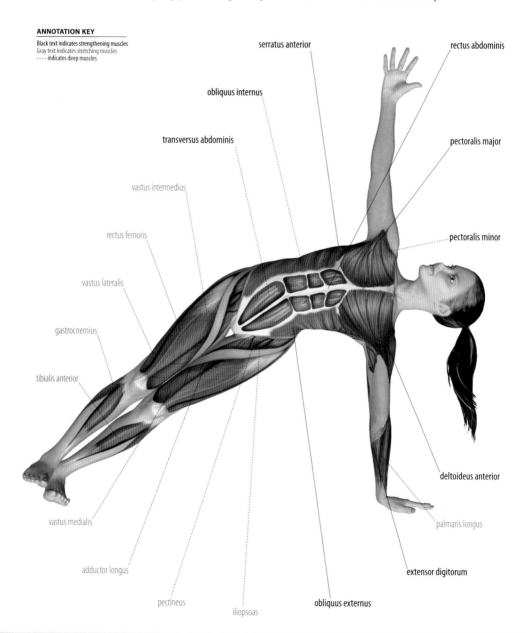

serratus anterior

rectus abdominis

obliquus internus

transversus abdominis

pectoralis major

vastus intermedius

rectus femoris

pectoralis minor

vastus lateralis

gastrocnemius

tibialis anterior

deltoideus anterior

vastus medialis

palmaris longus

adductor longus

extensor digitorum

pectineus

iliopsoas

obliquus externus

HOW TO DO IT

1 Begin in a plank position. Your arms should be straight with your wrists aligned under your shoulders.

2 Shift your weight onto the outside of your left foot and onto your left arm. Roll to the side, guiding with your hips and bringing your right shoulder back. Stack your right foot on top of the left, squeezing both legs together and straight.

3 Exhale, bring your right arm up toward the ceiling, and elongate your body, making a straight line from your head to your heels. Gaze up at your fingertips as you continue to push through your shoulder into the floor, maintaining a strong balance.

4 Keep breathing as you hold the position for 15 to 30 seconds. Release, and then repeat on the other side.

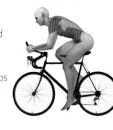

PRIMARY TARGETS
- rectus abdominis
- obliquus internus
- obliquus externus
- transversus abdominis
- pectoralis major
- pectoralis minor
- serratus anterior
- deltoideus anterior
- extensor digitorum

BENEFITS
- Strengthens abdominals, arms, legs, and wrists
- Improves balance

CAUTIONS
- Shoulder issues
- Wrist injury
- Elbow injury

PERFECT YOUR FORM
- Elongate your limbs as much as possible.
- Stack your flexed feet, as if they were side by side in standing position.
- Avoid allowing your hips or shoulders to sway or sink.
- Avoid lifting your hips too high.

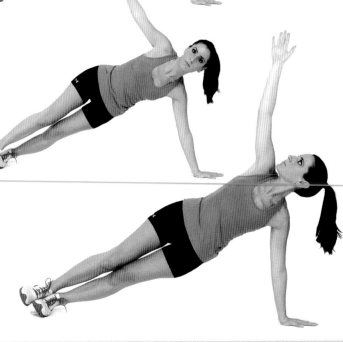

POWER SQUAT

ADVANCED

POWER SQUAT OFFERS a full-body workout that develops coordination and balance. With the benefits of both a squat and a deadlift to strengthen and tone your thighs and calves, it also calls for spinal rotation that works your back and obliques.

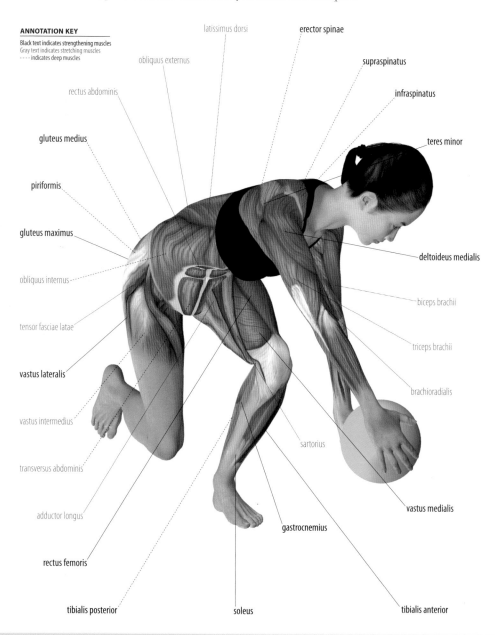

ANNOTATION KEY

Black text indicates strengthening muscles
Gray text indicates stretching muscles
- - - - indicates deep muscles

latissimus dorsi

erector spinae

obliquus externus

supraspinatus

rectus abdominis

infraspinatus

gluteus medius

teres minor

piriformis

gluteus maximus

deltoideus medialis

obliquus internus

biceps brachii

tensor fasciae latae

triceps brachii

vastus lateralis

brachioradialis

vastus intermedius

transversus abdominis

sartorius

adductor longus

vastus medialis

rectus femoris

gastrocnemius

tibialis posterior

soleus

tibialis anterior

HOW TO DO IT

1 Stand straight, holding a weighted medicine ball at shoulder height.

2 Shift your weight to your left foot, and bend your right knee, lifting your right foot toward your buttocks. Bend your elbows and draw the ball toward the outside of your right ear.

3 Maintaining a neutral spine, bend at your hips and knee. Lower your torso toward your left side, bringing the ball toward your left ankle.

4 Press into your left leg and straighten your knee and torso, returning to the starting position. Repeat 15 times for two sets on each leg.

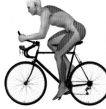

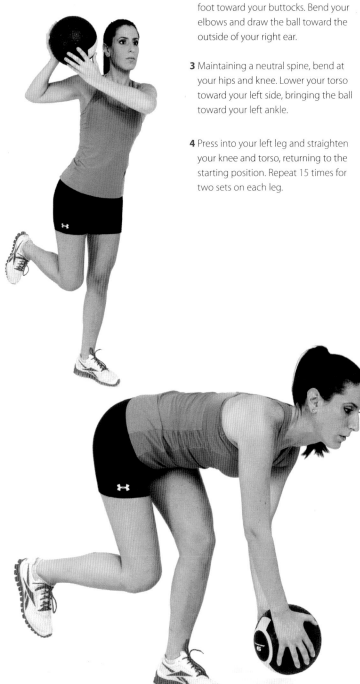

PRIMARY TARGETS
- vastus medialis
- vastus lateralis
- rectus femoris
- gluteus maximus
- gluteus medius
- piriformis
- erector spinae
- tibialis anterior
- tibialis posterior
- soleus
- gastrocnemius
- deltoideus medialis
- infraspinatus
- supraspinatus
- teres minor
- semitendinosus
- semimembranosus
- biceps femoris

BENEFITS
- Improves balance
- Stabilizes pelvis, trunk, and knees
- Promotes stronger movement patterns

CAUTIONS
- Knee pain
- Lower-back pain
- Shoulder pain

PERFECT YOUR FORM
- Keep your leading knee tight
- Avoid allowing your knee to extend beyond your toes as you bend and rotate.
- Avoid moving your standing foot from its starting position.
- Move the ball in an arc through the air.

IMPROVING YOUR POSTURE, BALANCE & COORDINATION

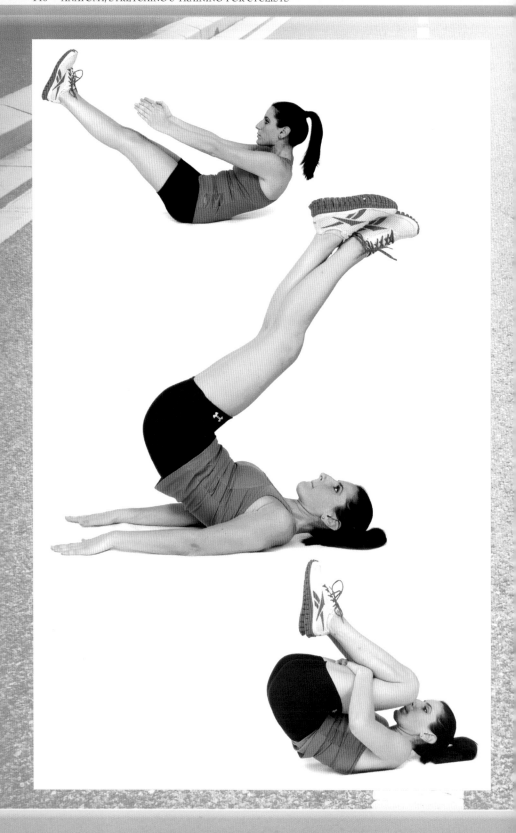

CYCLISTS' WORKOUTS

The following workouts have been devised with two purposes in mind: to help make you a better cyclist, and to keep your body balanced and in top shape.

It's now time to put together what you've learned throughout this book. Regardless of your fitness level, these workouts will benefit you. For instance, the Healthy Back Workout will help protect you from back fatigue on the bike, and the Balancing Workout will help develop muscles to stabilize your core.

Before stretching, be sure to warm up with some light cardio, whether this involves a brisk walk, a few jumping jacks, or some range-of-motion moves. Rest between exercises if necessary, and remember that the quality of your movement matters more than the number of repetitions you perform. Pay close attention to proper form, and you will find these workouts to be valuable, plateau-defeating tools in your progression to cycling fitness.

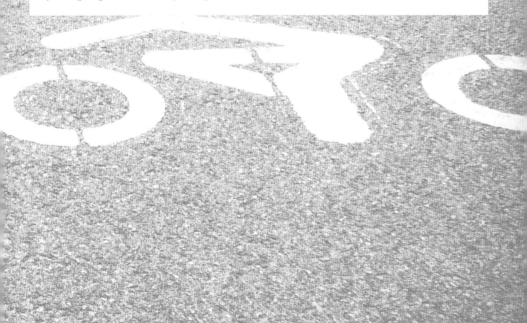

BEGINNER WORKOUT

Try these exercises either before or after a ride to stretch and tone your legs.

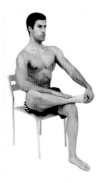

1 Point & Flex Foot Stretches
page 68

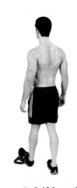

2 Calf Stretch
page 66

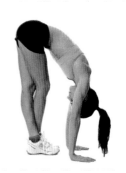

3 Iliotibial Band Stretch
page 52

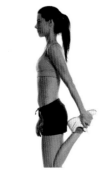

4 Standing Quads Stretch
page 56

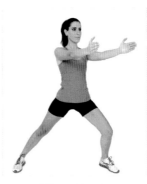

5 Lateral Low Lunge
page 80

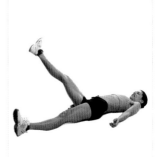

6 Unilateral Leg Circles
page 78

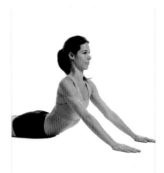

7 Cobra Stretch
page 40

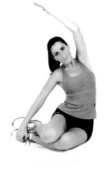

8 Side Mermaid
page 134

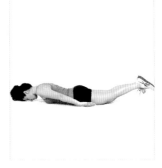

9 Heel Beats
page 84

INTERMEDIATE WORKOUT

Go to the next level with a workout that blends balance, strength, and flexibility exercises.

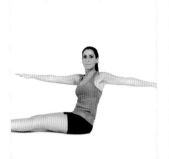

1 Spinal Twist
page 36

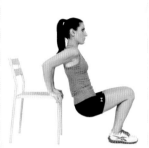

2 Chair Dip
page 72

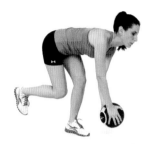

3 Power Squat
page 144

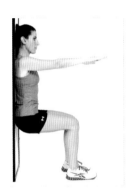

4 Wall Sit
page 86

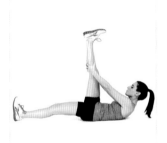

5 Scissors
page 102

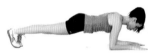

6 Plank Press-Up
page 92

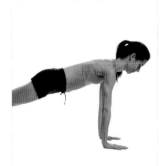

7 Push-Up
page 74

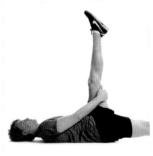

8 Unilateral Leg Raise
page 60

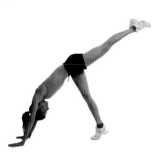

9 Three-Legged Dog
page 140

ADVANCED WORKOUT

Challenge yourself with a full-body workout for strength, posture, and flexibility.

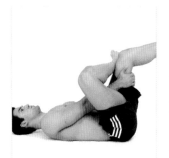

1 Supine Figure 4
page 42

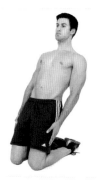

2 Thigh Rock-Back
page 100

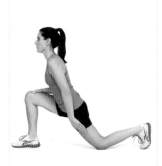

3 Hip Flexor Stretch
page 48

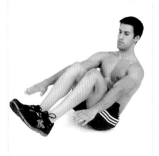

4 Lemon Squeezer
page 106

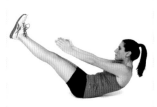

5 V-Up
page 118

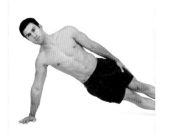

6 Side-Bend Plank
page 114

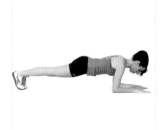

7 Plank Press-Up
page 90

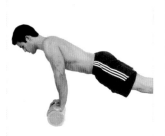

8 Foam Roller Push-Up
page 94

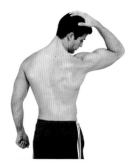

9 Trapezius Stretch
page 29

QUADRICEPS-STRENGTHENING WORKOUT

This series of exercises will help you begin building strength in the key running muscles.

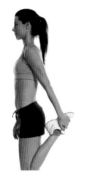

1 Standing Quads Stretch
page 56

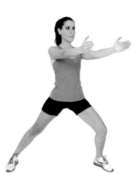

2 Lateral Low Lunge
page 80

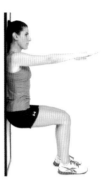

3 Wall Sit
page 86

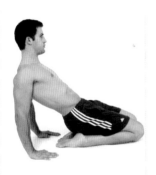

4 Shin Stretch
page 62

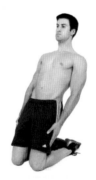

5 Thigh Rock-Back
page 100

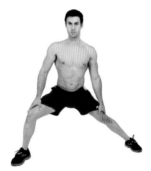

6 Hip Adductor Stretch
page 46

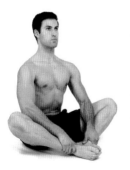

7 Butterfly Stretch
page 44

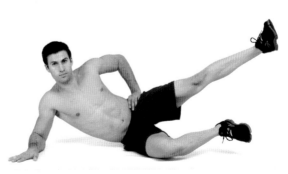

8 Clamshell Series
page 88

HEALTHY BACK WORKOUT

A strong back will help reduce fatigue during long rides, so work those muscles regularly.

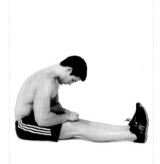

1 Lower & Upper Back Stretch
page 32

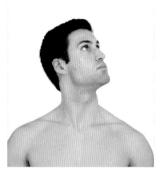

2 Cervical Stars
page 26

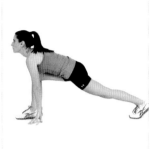

3 Yoga Lunge
page 82

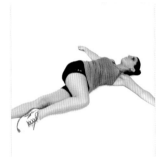

4 Spine Stretch
page 38

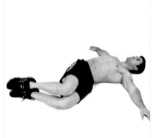

5 Lumbar Stretch
page 39

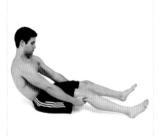

6 Scoop Rhomboids
page 33

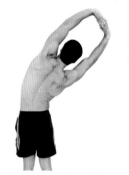

7 Latissimus Dorsi Stretch
page 34

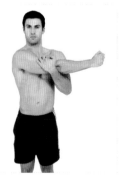

8 Shoulder Stretch
page 28

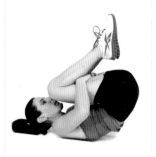

9 Rolling Like a Ball
page 130

CORE-STABILIZING WORKOUT

This series will help you achieve a strong, stable core that supports you on or off your bike.

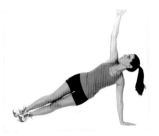

1 Side Plank Balance
page 142

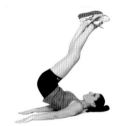

2 Abdominal Hip Lift
page 108

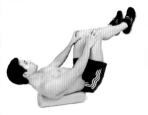

3 Foam Roller Dead Bug
page 120

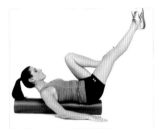

4 Foam Roller Bicycle
page 122

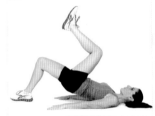

5 Bridge with Leg Lift
page 112

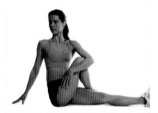

6 Hip/Iliotibial Band Stretch
page 50

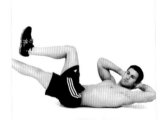

7 Crossover Crunch
page 104

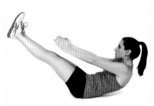

8 V-Up
page 118

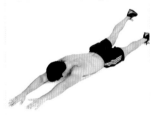

9 Swimming
page 128

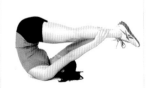

10 Open-Leg Rocker
page 138

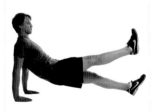

11 Front Plank Extension
page 116

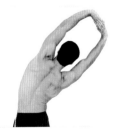

12 Latissimus Dorsi Stretch
page 34

LOW-IMPACT WORKOUT

For a low-impact workout that is easy on the joints, try this set of exercises.

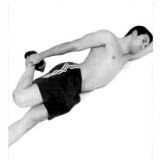

1 Side-Lying Knee Bend
page 58

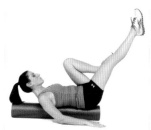

2 Foam Roller Bicycle
page 122

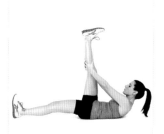

3 Scissors
page 102

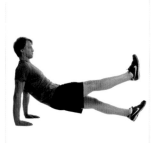

4 Front Plank Extension
page 116

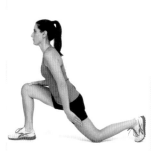

5 Hip Flexor Stretch
page 48

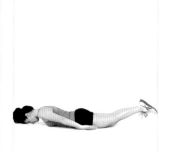

6 Heel Beats
page 84

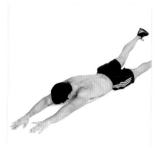

7 Swimming
page 128

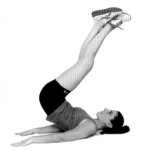

8 Abdominal Hip Lift
page 108

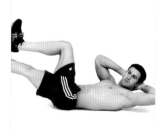

9 Crossover Crunch
page 104

STAMINA CHALLENGE

These challenging moves promote the stamina necessary for optimal cycling performance.

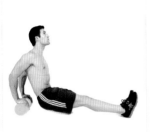

1 Foam Roller Triceps Dip
page 96

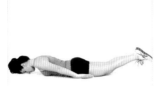

2 Heel Beats
page 84

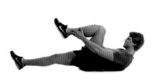

3 Abdominal Kick
page 110

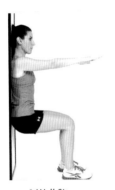

4 Wall Sit
page 86

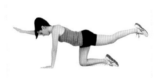

5 Quadruped Leg Lift
page 126

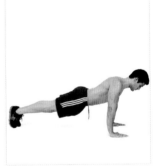

6 Plank Roll-Down
page 90

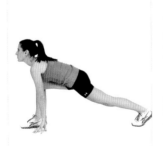

7 Yoga Lunge
page 82

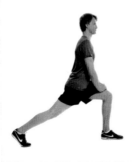

8 Forward Lunge
page 54

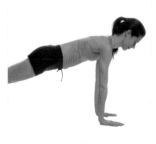

9 Push-Up
page 74

BALANCING WORKOUT

This set of exercises will help you hone your sense of balance—a cycling necessity.

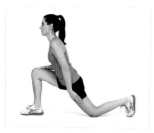

1 Hip Flexor Stretch
page 48

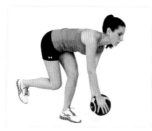

2 Power Squat
page 144

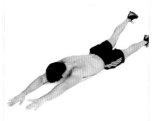

3 Swimming
page 128

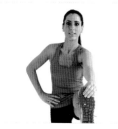

4 Hand-to-Toe Lift
page 64

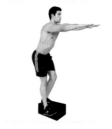

5 Step-Down
page 76

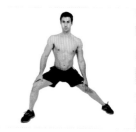

6 Hip Adductor Stretch
page 46

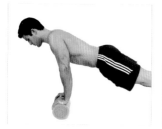

7 Foam Roller Push-Up
page 94

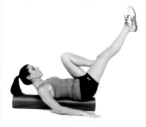

8 Foam Roller Bicycle
page 122

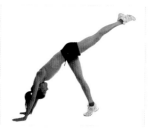

9 Three-Legged Dog
page 140

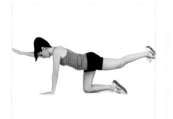

10 Quadruped Leg Lift
page 126

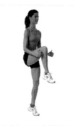

11 Standing Knee Crunch
page 136

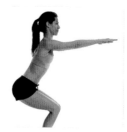

12 Knee Squat
page 132

POSTURAL WORKOUT

To develop good posture on and off your bike, try this set of targeted exercises.

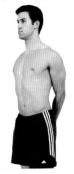

1 Chest Stretch
page 30

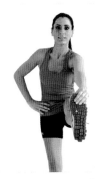

2 Hand-to-Toe Lift
page 64

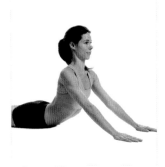

3 Cobra Stretch
page 40

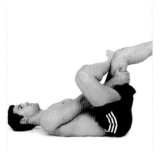

4 Supine Figure 4
page 42

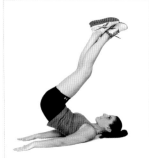

5 Abdominal Hip Lift
page 108

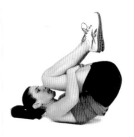

6 Rolling Like a Ball
page 130

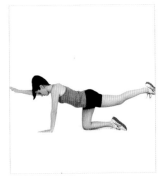

7 Quadruped Leg Lift
page 126

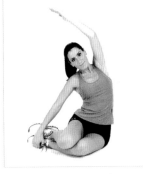

8 Side Mermaid
page 134

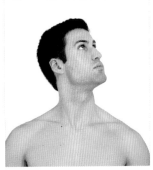

9 Cervical Stars
page 26

GLOSSARY OF MUSCULATURE

The following glossary explains the Latin scientific terminology used to describe the muscles of the human body. Certain words are derived from Greek, which is indicated in each instance.

CHEST

coracobrachialis: Greek *korakoeidés*, 'ravenlike,' and *brachium*, 'arm'

pectoralis (major and minor): *pectus*, 'breast'

ABDOMEN

obliquus externus: *obliquus*, 'slanting,' and *externus*, 'outward'

obliquus internus: *obliquus*, 'slanting,' and *internus*, 'within'

rectus abdominis: *rego*, 'straight, upright,' and *abdomen*, 'belly'

serratus anterior: *serra*, 'saw,' and *ante*, 'before'

transversus abdominis: *transversus*, 'athwart,' and *abdomen*, 'belly'

NECK

scalenus: Greek *skalénós*, 'unequal'

semispinalis: *semi*, 'half,' and *spinae*, 'spine'

splenius: Greek *spléníon*, 'plaster, patch'

sternocleidomastoideus: Greek *stérnon*, 'chest,' Greek *kleís*, 'key' and Greek *mastoeidés*, 'breastlike'

BACK

erector spinae: *erectus*, 'straight,' and *spina*, 'thorn'

latissimus dorsi: *latus*, 'wide,' and *dorsum*, 'back'

multifidus spinae: *multifid*, 'to cut into divisions,' and *spinae*, 'spine'

quadratus lumborum: *quadratus*, 'square, rectangular,' and *lumbus*, 'loin'

rhomboideus: Greek *rhembesthai*, 'to spin'

trapezius: Greek *trapezion*, 'small table'

SHOULDERS

deltoideus (anterior, medial, and posterior): Greek *deltoeidés*, 'delta-shaped'

infraspinatus: *infra*, 'under,' and *spina*, 'thorn'

levator scapulae: *levare*, 'to raise,' and *scapulae*, 'shoulder [blades]'

subscapularis: *sub*, 'below,' and *scapulae*, 'shoulder [blades]'

supraspinatus: *supra*, 'above,' and *spina*, 'thorn'

teres (major and minor): *teres*, 'rounded'

UPPER ARM

biceps brachii: *biceps*, 'two-headed,' and *brachium*, 'arm'

brachialis: *brachium*, 'arm'

triceps brachii: *triceps*, 'three-headed,' and *brachium*, 'arm'

LOWER ARM

anconeus: Greek *anconad*, 'elbow'

brachioradialis: *brachium*, 'arm,' and *radius*, 'spoke'

extensor carpi radialis: *extendere*, 'to extend,' Greek *karpós*, 'wrist', and *radius*, 'spoke'

extensor digitorum: *extendere*, 'to extend,' and *digitus*, 'finger, toe'

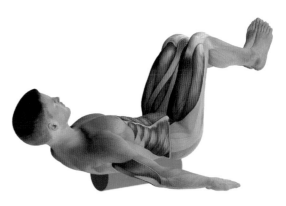

flexor carpi pollicis longus: *flectere*, 'to bend', Greek *karpós*, 'wrist', *pollicis*, 'thumb', and *longus*, 'long'

flexor carpi radialis: *flectere*, 'to bend', Greek *karpós*, 'wrist', and *radius*, 'spoke'

flexor carpi ulnaris: *flectere*, 'to bend', Greek *karpós*, 'wrist', and *ulnaris*, 'forearm'

flexor digitorum: *flectere*, 'to bend', and *digitus*, 'finger, toe'

palmaris longus: *palmaris*, 'palm', and *longus*, 'long'

pronator teres: *pronate*, 'to rotate', and *teres*, 'rounded'

HIPS

gemellus (inferior and superior): *geminus*, 'twin'

gluteus maximus: Greek *gloutós*, 'rump', and *maximus*, 'largest'

gluteus medius: Greek *gloutós*, 'rump', and *medialis*, 'middle'

gluteus minimus: Greek *gloutós*, 'rump', and *minimus*, 'smallest'

iliopsoas: *ilium*, 'groin', and Greek *psoa*, 'groin muscle'

obturator externus: *obturare*, 'to block', and *externus*, 'outward'

obturator internus: *obturare*, 'to block', and *internus*, 'within'

pectineus: *pectin*, 'comb'

piriformis: *pirum*, 'pear', and *forma*, 'shape'

quadratus femoris: *quadratus*, 'square, rectangular', and *femur*, 'thigh'

UPPER LEG

adductor longus: *adducere*, 'to contract', and *longus*, 'long'

adductor magnus: *adducere*, 'to contract', and *magnus*, 'major'

biceps femoris: *biceps*, 'two-headed', and *femur*, 'thigh'

gracilis: *gracilis*, 'slim, slender'

rectus femoris: *rego*, 'straight, upright', and *femur*, 'thigh'

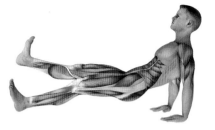

sartorius: *sarcio*, 'to patch' or 'to repair'

semimembranosus: *semi*, 'half', and *membrum*, 'limb'

semitendinosus: *semi*, 'half', and *tendo*, 'tendon'

tensor fasciae latae: *tenere*, 'to stretch', *fasciae*, 'band', and *latae*, 'laid down'

vastus intermedius: *vastus*, 'immense, huge', and *intermedius*, 'between'

vastus lateralis: *vastus*, 'immense, huge', and *lateralis*, 'side'

vastus medialis: *vastus*, 'immense, huge', and *medialis*, 'middle'

LOWER LEG

adductor digiti minimi: *adducere*, 'to contract', *digitus*, 'finger, toe', and *minimum* 'smallest'

adductor hallucis: *adducere*, 'to contract', and *hallex*, 'big toe'

extensor digitorum longus: *extendere*, 'to extend', *digitus*, 'finger, toe', and *longus*, 'long'

extensor hallucis longus: *extendere*, 'to extend', *hallex*, 'big toe', and *longus*, 'long'

flexor digitorum longus: *flectere*, 'to bend', *digitus*, 'finger, toe', and *longus*, 'long'

flexor hallucis longus: *flectere*, 'to bend', and *hallex*, 'big toe', and *longus*, 'long'

gastrocnemius: Greek *gastroknémía*, 'calf [of the leg]'

peroneus: *peronei*, 'of the fibula'

plantaris: *planta*, 'the sole'

soleus: *solea*, 'sandal'

tibialis anterior: *tibia*, 'reed pipe', and *ante*, 'before'

tibialis posterior: *tibia*, 'reed pipe', and *posterus*, 'coming after'

CREDITS

Created by Lisa Purcell Editorial & Design for Moseley Road Inc.

Moseley Road Inc.
123 Main Street
Irvington, New York 10533

President: Sean Moore
Production director: Adam Moore
Project art and editorial director: Lisa Purcell

Editor: Erica Gordon-Mallin

Contributing writers: Amy Auman and Lisa Purcell

Photographers: FineArtsPhotoGroup.com and Jonathan Conklin Photography, Inc.

Model: David Anderson, Maria Grippi, Sara Blowers, and Nicolay Alexandrov

Illustrator: Hector Aiza/3D Labz Animation India (www.3dlabz.com)

Photographs by FineArtsPhotoGroup.com, except pages 41 (bottom box), 51–57, 61, 75, 79, 111, 117, 127 (box), 133, 137, 141, 148 (top row right), 148 (middle row left), 148 (bottom row left), 140 (bottom row, left, center, right), 151 (top row left), 153 (second row right), 153 (bottom row center), 154 (middle row left), 155 (top row right), 155 (bottom row center, right), 156 (third row right), 156 (bottom row center, right), 157 (top row right) by Jonathan Conklin Photography, Inc.; and pages 8 Stefan Schurr/Shutterstock.com; 11 Ikonoklast Fotografie/Shutterstock.com; 12 sainthorant daniel/Shutterstock.com; 13 (left) titov dmitriy; 13 (right) Diego Cervo/Shutterstock.com; 14 jo Crebbin/Shutterstock.com; 15 Toddy1979/Shutterstock.com; 16 Warren Goldswain/Shutterstock.com; 17 (left) Mike Flippo/Shutterstock.com; 17 (top right) Robyn Mackenzie/Shutterstock.com; 17 (bottom right) Feng Yu/Shutterstock.com; 18 (top) FineArtsPhotoGroup.com; 18 (bottom) Tatuasha/Shutterstock.com; 19 Monkey Business Images/Shutterstock.com; 20 melis/Shutterstock.com; 21 steamroller_blues/Shutterstock.com.

Anatomical illustrations by Hector Aiza except pages 22 and 23 by Linda Bucklin/Shutterstock.com.

ABOUT THE AUTHOR

Lisa Purcell is a New York City book designer, editor, and writer. A graduate of Princeton University, she specializes in health and fitness books.